D0217213

Sexual Health Concerns: Interviewing and History Taking for Health Practitioners

Michael W. Ross

MA MHPEd MPH DipTertEd DipSTD PhD CPsychol FBPsS FRSH

WHO Center for Health Promotion Research and Development
School of Public Health
University of Texas at Houston

Lorna D. Channon-Little

MSc PhD MBPS

Department of Behavioural Science in Medicine
The University of Sydney

B.R. Simon Rosser

MA PhD MPH LP

Program in Human Sexuality
Department of Family Practice and Community Health,
Medical School
University of Minnesota

SETON HALL UNIVERSITY
UNIVERSITY LIBRARIES
SO. ORANGE. NJ 07079-2671

 F. A. DAVIS COMPANY • Philadelphia

For Geoffrey and Leo
For Rafael

First published 1991 as Discussing Sexuality: A Guide for health practitioners

Second edition 2000
Reprinted 2000

F. A. Davis Company
1915 Arch Street
Philadelphia, PA 19103

©2000 MacLennan & Petty Pty Limited

All rights reserved. This book is protected by copyright. No part of it may be reproduced, stored in a retrieval system, or transmitted in any form or by any means, electronic, mechanical, photocopying, recording, or otherwise, without written permission from the publisher.

Cataloging-in-Publication Data
This information is available from the Library of Congress
ISBN 0-8036-0668-0

Authorization to photocopy items for internal or personal use, or the internal or personal use of specific clients, is granted by F.A. Davis Company for users registered with the Copyright Clearance Centre (CCC) Transactional Reporting Service, provided that the fee of $.10 per copy is paid directly to CCC, 222 Rosewood Drive, Salem, MA 01923. For those organizations that have been granted a photocopy license by CCC, a separate system of payment has been arranged. The fee code for users of the Transactional Reporting Service is: 8036-0414/99 0 + $.10.

Printed and bound in Singapore

HQ
60.5
·R68
2000

Contents

Foreword 1   v

Foreword 2   viii

Acknowledgments   x

Preface   xi

1.   Introduction: Why take a sexual history?   1

2.   How to take a sexual history   7

3.   Taking a sexual history   23

4.   Sexual history taking for sexually transmissible diseases   40

5.   Sexual counselling   51

6.   Sexual counselling and treatment   57

7.   Reactions to STD infection and STD counselling   87

8.   Sexuality and preventive health care   113

9.   Sexuality and chronic illness   120

10. Sexuality and drug-related history   126

11. Pre-test and post-test HIV counselling   130

12. Legal and ethical considerations   151

13. Understanding and counselling sexual orientation
     concerns   161

14. Sexual counselling of children and adolescents   182

15. Sexuality and aging   205

Index   216

Foreword 1

In more than twenty years of teaching human sexuality to medical students, physicians and other health care providers, I continue to find that the most difficult issue is to develop the comfort and ability of the health care professional to discuss sexuality with their patients. This is an essential ingredient in providing optimal sexual health care. While there is more openness in discussing sexuality in our culture today, many health care professionals still find it uncomfortable to talk about sexuality in an open and comfortable manner. Yet, in order to provide optimal health care, the health care professional needs to be comfortable and knowledgeable in discussing sexuality and sexual health concerns with patients. These are issues that health care providers will encounter on a daily basis and they need the tools to address them.

Many of us grew up in environments where sex and sexuality were forbidden topics or were the topics of joking or teasing. Consequently, patients and health care professionals alike may not always feel comfortable discussing these matters in a clinical setting. Even those professionals who are comfortable discussing sexuality in their private lives are often concerned about upsetting patients by asking sexual questions. Rarely do health care professionals acknowledge their own discomfort and lack of knowledge. In my experience, they often project their anxiety onto the patient. However, many patients have sexual problems and concerns and want their health care provider to bring up the topic.

The problem has been and continues to be the inadequate training that professionals are given. Most health care providers have never received an effective lecture as part of their professional training on 'Taking a Sex History.' While some professionals have received human sexuality lectures or have had specific courses in human sexuality and sexual health care, rarely has there been an emphasis on the practical tools of asking questions about sexuality, diagnosing a sexual problem or disorder, brief treatment approaches, and reasons for referral.

And yet without this training, the health care professional is usually the first point of contact for individuals with sexual concerns and problems. Patients naturally expect competence and a nonjudgmental attitude from their health care provides. Patients don't expect their providers to know everything, but they do expect and appreciate careful listening and caring.

The primary job of any health care professional is to identify problems and concerns and try to alleviate them. With a greater emphasis on prevention in health care today, health care providers are also required to identify risk factors in order to prevent problems from occurring or recurring. There are many ways that the health care professional can be helpful. Many times, sexual problems and concerns can be alleviated and prevented by careful listening, compassion, debunking of myths, and providing basic information. Providing accurate information about sexuality can help patients understand their own sexual developmental process or identify problems of concern if they do occur. We also know that many of the sexual problems in couples are rooted in poor communication about sexuality. The health care professional can be a role-model of healthy communication. Helping a patient understand how their illness or medication may be affecting their sexual functioning can relieve many anxieties and concerns. If these approaches do not resolve the concern, the health care professional can search more for underlying physical or psychological causes for their distress. Some problems need further medical or psychological intervention. Today, we have a much greater understanding of the biomedical aspects of sexual functioning and dysfunction. New biomedical treatments have been developed. Altering medications or using medications which might assist in improving sexual functioning can be very helpful. In other cases, referral to specialists, including sexual therapists is needed. Ultimately, as health care professionals, we all can offer compassion, understanding and hope to those who need help.

To some health care providers, counselling patients can seem like a mysterious and time-consuming endeavor. This book illustrates some simple and brief counselling interventions which can be very helpful. I try to encourage health care providers to learn these techniques and use them with their patients. I find that when the health care provider has developed enough of a therapeutic relationship with the patient to discuss these matters then the provider is in a good position to provide the counselling. Not only is a positive outcome possible, but the process of counselling enhances the therapeutic relationship—which is of benefit to both the patient and the provider.

I always found the first edition of this book to be extremely helpful in teaching human sexuality to health care providers. This updated edition retains the concise and helpful format of the first one with up-to-date information and some excellent new chapters on counselling children and adolescents and dealing with sexuality and aging.

This book provides an excellent and practical approach to effective sexual health care. In a step-by-step fashion, the reader is given practical approaches to discussing sexuality and sexual health concerns with their patients. The reader is given very practical tips on subjects from asking basic screening questions to completing more detailed sexual histories. Examples of helpful, probing questions are given which can help identify common sexual concerns, dysfunctions and disorders.

As sexuality is such an integral part of a person, sexual health is essential to one's overall health and well being. Every person, no matter what their age, ethnicity, religion, gender, sexual orientation, physical condition, illness or disability will have sexual questions and may have some concerns or problems sometime in their lifetime. By reading this book, health care professionals will be able to better address these critical issues in the context of providing optimal and comprehensive health care.

ELI COLEMAN *PhD*
Professor and Director
Program in Human Sexuality
University of Minnesota Medical School
Minneapolis, January 1999

Foreword 2

Medical students do not like to listen to people. In this they are no different from established practitioners who too often do not like to listen either. Actually, people generally do not like to listen. They like to talk—most of all, about themselves! Medical practitioners are ready to talk, ready to give advice, ready to counsel, but they are not good listeners. Just ask Australian Aborigines—they will tell you that white Australians are not good listeners generally and it is likely that a wider group of people do not listen well either.

Yet the taking of a history is where clinical encounters begin and it is active, intelligent listening that allows the practitioner to gain most from that meeting. It is not only medical practitioners who are aware that non-verbal cues are significant; patients are aware too. If the signal sent non-verbally does not match other messages, the non-verbal communication is believed and the other messages are ignored. Good history taking increases the chance the patient will gain benefit from the encounter; poor history taking reduces the chance of that benefit occurring.

For many practitioners and patients the taking of a sexual history is traumatic. It involves intruding into areas of private activity, asking embarrassing questions, seeking language on sensitive matters which is clear to both parties, seeking an extension of trust often not available to anyone else. While questions may concern sexual diseases, they can as easily concern relationships and usual sexual functioning.

We teach the newest of our students about communication, about how to listen, about how to see and hear the messages that people send. Later in the course we teach Health Ethics and Law so that students have some idea of the ethical context within which much clinical activity occurs. And all this before the students have really studied clinical medicine.

The culture of hospitals does not value privacy, confidentiality, patient autonomy, beneficence or justice. Yet these 'principles', flawed as they might be theoretically, are the touchstones we give to young men and women about to enter medical practice. The messages our young colleagues receive from hospitals do not prepare them well for community practice. Actually, the whole culture of medicine tends too much to be disease-directed and not enough to be person-directed.

This book empowers practitioners. It teaches something of the content of the sexual history (and may be almost alone in so doing) but additionally it helps practitioners feel more easy about the interaction, about the exchange, about the duties we take on, and about how we might be of most use to those consulting us. If the quality of the history is important for the outcome, we can all be better practitioners by learning some of the lessons this book teaches.

We are deeply in the debt of these authors. They have helped us to become better practitioners in an area that is becoming more important and more relevant. We can only be assisted by an excellent book like this one.

PETER BAUME *AO*
Head
School of Community Medicine
University of New South Wales
Sydney, April 1999

Acknowledgments

The second edition of this book would not have been possible without help from a number of sources. In particular, we wish to acknowledge the assistance of Professor Eli Coleman, PhD, for helpful suggestions on improving the manuscript and sexual history questions. We also acknowledge Ms Anne-Marie Weber Main at the University of Minnesota for her assistance in editing the manuscript. Adis International Limited kindly consented to allow us to reproduce modified versions of several papers in *Patient Management* as sections of chapters. These include the following:

Ross, M.W. Counselling the homosexual patient. *Patient Management*, 1983; 7(7): 117–123.

Ross, M.W. Understanding the homosexual patient. *Patient Management*, 1985; 9: 15–25.

Ross, M.W. and Rosser, B.R.S. Pretest counselling for AIDS screening: a guide for the clinician. *Patient Management*, 1987; 11(7): 93–103.

Ross, M.W. and Rosser, B.R.S. Counselling the patient with an STD. *Patient Management*, 1988; 17(8): 73–84.

Ross, M.W. Principles of patient counselling. *Viral Therapy in General Practice*, 1989; 4: 1–3.

Any errors in the text, however, are solely the responsibility of the authors.

Preface

We have always assumed that such a basic necessity as a book on sexual history taking and counselling would be not only readily available but also a common text in medical and nursing courses. Therefore our first response on being asked to write such a book in 1991 was: why write another one? On attempting to find such texts we were surprised that there was little available, and what was available was either too specialized or too brief. Why was there so little material on such an important area?

As we were teachers in medical schools as well as clinicians, and as we teach human sexuality to medical students, we were acutely aware of the need for adequate training in the area not only of human sexuality, but the practical skills necessary to take a history, make a diagnosis, formulate a treatment plan or make an appropriate referral. The advent of HIV/AIDS in the last decades together with increased public awareness and discussion of STDs such as herpes, gonorrhea, chlamydia and syphilis, and pelvic inflammatory disease, in the last few years has meant that practitioners are more likely to be asked about STDs by their patients. Indeed, they are expected to be comfortable in discussing sexuality and STDs. However, our encounters with students and colleagues suggested that while most recognized the need, few had the skills necessary or were comfortable in taking a sexual history. This was not helped by the pressure of time in medical and nursing courses as a result of the increased complexity of medical science and technology. Nevertheless, we believe that the art of health practice is still as important as the science, particularly in an area as relatively neglected as sexuality.

On being asked to write a second edition in 1998, we were disturbed to note that the need is still as great as it was in 1991: if anything, the gap between the patient or client's awareness and the ability of the practitioner to address it has widened. Despite the increase in programs teaching health professionals the basic skills to make them competent to approach sexual health issues in their patients or clients, there have also been losses, for example the withdrawal of such programs, or making them optional—which is often preaching to the converted.

In response to these perceived needs we wrote this book as a manual rather than as a text. In doing so we recognize that a substantial number of practitioners will have had no training in the area. Even more will have had only introductory exposure to human sexuality during their training. Therefore we have tried to combine the steps necessary to take a sexual history and make a diagnosis in as simple a form as possible giving the reasons for each step. This book is unashamedly aimed at the practitioner and does not attempt to create experts in sexual therapy. Rather, we are hoping to enhance the basic skills of practitioners in what has become an integral part of health practice. We hope that it will prove useful as a guide to sexual history taking and counselling for practitioners who feel the need to expand or refresh their clinical skills.

MICHAEL W. ROSS (Houston)
LORNA D. CHANNON-LITTLE (Sydney)
B.R. SIMON ROSSER (Minneapolis)
January 1999

1 Introduction: Why take a sexual history?

In the last few decades, the subject of human sexuality has become a topic of intense debate in society. Particularly in the printed and electronic media, discussions about sexuality are an almost daily occurrence. Advertisements for condoms appear on prime-time television. Television and radio talk-show hosts examine sexual topics, including sexual minority concerns, STDs and HIV, advances in sexual medicine, and a plethora of sex-related issues. On the Internet, intense discussion about sex and censorship transcends national boundaries. Even the inquiry into the sex life of President Clinton and other politicians has led to public discussions of such previously taboo topics as oral sex, extramarital affairs, sexual abuse and the meaning of consensual sexual conduct. Clearly, the general public perceives sex as a subject suitable for discussion and is probably now better informed about this subject than at any other time in western history.

Advances in sexuality research have also increased the public's knowledge about common and uncommon sexual behaviors. People are more concerned about sexual performance, and also more willing to seek help for sexual problems. With the advent of new treatments for sexual functioning, such as Viagra, more patients are discussing their sexual concerns with their health practitioners. In addition, the prevalence of sexually transmissible diseases (STDs) including gonorrhea, syphilis, genital herpes, human papilloma virus, hepatitis B and C, chlamydia and human immunodeficiency virus (HIV) has made it likely that most practitioners will be faced with the task of taking a sexual history and engaging in some form of sexual counselling.

Unfortunately, despite the courses on sexuality in schools of medicine, nursing, social work, public health and psychology (courses that range from the token to the thorough), many health practitioners remain uncomfortable about or relatively untrained in taking sexual histories, diagnosing sexual problems and counselling patients with sexual concerns. Even while more and more science and technology is being fitted into courses for health practitioners, areas such as sexual history taking and the diagnosis of sexual problems tend to be underemphasized. Even if the basic skills exist, discomfort with the area of sexuality can discourage health practitioners from broaching the subject with their patients.[1]

The aim of this book is to provide a simple, straightforward guide for the health practitioner: the why, how, when and where of taking a sexual history, with sufficient detail about sexual dysfunctions and behaviors to allow the practitioner to make a basic diagnosis and either carry out appropriate counselling or make a suitable referral. This book comprises three areas: how to take a sexual history; how to diagnose sexual dysfunctions; and how to undertake basic sexual counselling.

REASONS FOR BEING SKILLED IN TAKING A SEXUAL HISTORY

There are a number of good reasons why taking competent sexual histories is a necessary skill for the health practitioner. First, the health practitioner is usually the point of first contact for the person with a sexual dysfunction or sexually transmissible disease (STD). Failure to seriously and professionally treat the person or the presenting problem will neither resolve the problem nor enhance the reputation of the practitioner. If particular health practitioners do not meet the sexual health needs of their patients, then it is likely that people will consult others who do. Particularly in urban areas with a wide choice of practitioners, the inability of certain practitioners to offer particular services or to deal comfortably with the full range of presenting problems may be one of a number of factors that lead people to shop around for their health care.

Second, patients and clients clearly expect the health practitioner to have some knowledge of sexual health issues. The great majority of both adolescents and adults believe that the health practitioner is the most appropriate person to approach for problems with sexual dysfunctions, questions about sexuality, or STDs. While specialists from a number of other professions treat sexual dysfunctions or STDs, it is expected that the practitioner will at a minimum take a history, make a diagnosis, offer appropriate advice and either refer or counsel the patient or client themselves.

Third, as we have already noted, sex has become a topic of discussion in newspapers and magazines, on radio and television, and even in social conversation. As a result, people are more concerned about sexual problems, more aware of the risks of STDs, and more willing to ask questions or seek help. The incidence of asking about sexual matters has risen markedly since

1960, initially as a result of an increase in use of contraceptives such as the anovulant pill, and more recently spurred on by greater awareness of STDs (of which herpes and HIV are probably the best known).

Sexual dysfunctions and STDs are not uncommon, and it will be rare for the practitioner in the community not to see several potential cases per year. We use the term 'potential' because if the practitioner doesn't ask about problems, they are usually not discovered. Health practitioners differ with regard to their estimates of the proportion of their patients who have sexual difficulties: surgeons estimate the proportion to be as low as 15%, psychiatrists suggest it may be as high as 70%. While these figures may also reflect the different types of patients seen, even if one in seven patients may have a sexual problem the average practitioner may need to take at least one sexual history per day. In addition to the prevalence of sexual dysfunctions, the AIDS epidemic has focussed attention on counselling associated with STDs. In some areas, testing for HIV requires mandatory (by law) pre- and post-test counselling. It is often impractical to refer on to a counsellor unless the practitioner is associated with a specialized STD or AIDS clinic, so taking a sexual history and counselling is a much more common requirement.

In spite of the increased freedom to discuss sexual matters, people remain in doubt about many aspects of sexuality. The Kinsey Institute receives 'thousands of letters and telephone calls from people seeking accurate, up-to-date answers to questions about sex' each year, and in its Report even entitled one of the chapters 'America fails sex information test'.[2]

Fourth, the role of health practitioners has changed. Now, a greater emphasis is placed on primary prevention and health education, and a significant proportion of this relates to sexual matters. For women, areas where the health practitioner should advise and educate the patient include the need for regular Pap smears to detect cervical cancer, the choice of an appropriate contraceptive for the woman's lifestyle and the monitoring of its use, screening for breast cancer (including mammography), and the possibility of pelvic inflammatory disease (PID). For men, as for women, the possibility of subclinical STD infection, and advice on appropriate prophylaxis such as condoms, are important aspects of preventive health care, as is advice to young men about regular examination for testicular cancer.

Finally, the widespread public response in terms of prescription requests to the availability of Viagra alerted us to the fact that erectile dysfunction may have been more widespread than was assumed. Alternatively, it may also have been an indication of the reluctance of patients to raise the issue with practitioners until an efficacious treatment was available. Recent

3

evidence[3] from a large random sample of over 3,000 US adults in 1992 suggests that sexual dysfunctions are more widespread than was previously thought.

In women, 30% reported lack of interest in sex (this was higher in African American women and in those with lower education), around 25% were unable to achieve orgasm (more common in the never married and divorced), and around 15% experienced pain during sex (more common in younger women). Finding sex unpleasurable was reported by one in five women (it was more common in younger women), while performance anxiety was reported by about one in eight (again, more common in younger women). Trouble lubricating was reported by one in five women.

In men, around 15% reported lack of interest in sex (more common in older men, the never married, and in the divorced, separated or widowed group), although less than 10% reported being unable to achieve orgasm. Climaxing too early (premature ejaculation) was reported by 30% of men, with no significant demographic predictors, while trouble maintaining or achieving an erection was reported by the same proportion. Nearly 20% reported being anxious about their sexual performance, while less than 10% reported that sex was not pleasurable.

Of particular interest was the fact that Laumann and colleagues found that emotional problems and stress were significantly associated with low desire or arousal disorder in women, and with premature ejaculation, erectile dysfunction, and low desire in men. Low physical sexual satisfaction, low emotional satisfaction, and low general happiness were all significantly associated with all classes of sexual dysfunction (with the exception of premature ejaculation in men). Whether measuring cause or effect, these findings underscore the distress and marital disturbance associated with sexual dysfunction and the importance of taking a sexual history where marital discord is apparent.

Taken together, these figures indicate that sexual dysfunction will affect at least one third of the adult population in the United States, and we have no reason to assume that this figure would differ in similar western societies. The low estimates of sexual dysfunction and the lack of relevant clinical enquiry by health practitioners may be an indicator of professional discomfort rather than anything else. The figures which Laumann and colleagues[3] report suggest that sexual dysfunction is one of the more common difficulties experienced in the US adult population, and that a lack of enquiry from a health practitioner would be hard to justify on medical, psychological or epidemiological grounds.

REASONS WHY MOST HEALTH PRACTITIONERS ARE NOT ABLE TO TAKE A GOOD SEXUAL HISTORY

Many health practitioners are unskilled or uncomfortable in taking a sexual history. The general lack of adequate instruction in sexuality, and lack of opportunities for practice in taking sexual histories which would normally desensitize the practitioner's discomfort, means that practitioners out in the community may need to enhance their skills before they are comfortable taking a sexual history. Comfort comes for the practitioner with both practice and a sense of control over the subject, and this comfort is communicated to the patient. Conversely, when both the practitioner and the patient are embarrassed, they may attempt to skirt around the subject, resulting in inadequate or inaccurate histories and diagnoses subject to greater uncertainty or error. This will also ensure that sexual problems are not raised in the future.

Merrill and colleagues[4] identified three major reasons why practitioners fail to take adequate sexual histories: embarrassment, a belief that a sexual history is not relevant to the patient's chief complaint, and the fact that practitioners are not adequately trained. In a survey of senior medical students in the United States, Merrill and colleagues found that while 93% thought that knowledge of a patient's sexual practices was an important part of their patient's medical history, half felt poorly trained to take such a history, and a quarter felt embarrassed to ask the necessary questions.

A number of personal characteristics were found to be related to difficulties in taking a sexual history.[4] Those who were most shy and socially anxious were most likely to feel embarrassment, while an unsympathetic view of a patient's psychological problems was most closely related to the belief that the sexual history was of little importance in understanding a patient's problem. The sense of not feeling adequately trained to take a sexual history related most strongly to lower self-esteem. These data suggest that the difficulties in taking a sexual history, while common, can be overcome with training and experience.

In summary, there are a number of compelling reasons why the health practitioner should be sufficiently competent to take at the minimum a sexual history, if not to engage in basic sexual counselling. Even if the decision is to refer, it is not possible to write an adequate referral without having taken a sexual history. And without a sexual history, it is not possible to determine whether the referral should be to a psychologist, psychiatrist, endocrinologist, neurologist, urologist, gynaecologist, marriage counsellor, general sex therapist, social worker, or another appropriate professional.

If the presenting problem has STD as a possible diagnosis, then basic examination cannot take place without the practitioner taking a sexual history to determine what sites should be investigated and the probable latency of infection, which will make differential diagnosis possible. The sexual history is a subset of a general history, and taking a history is probably the most basic and most essential skill of the health practitioner today. So while the content of a sexual history may differ from that of a general history, the practice of taking the history is neither a totally new skill, nor one peripheral to modern clinical practice. There are various opinions as to when to take a sexual history, but not as to its importance. Lief[5] puts it this way:

> The vast number of problems that involve aspects of sexual functioning, the increase in the demand for services, and the expectation of patients that the health practitioner be competent and skilful in the management of sexual problems create a situation in which there is no real choice. The health practitioner must learn the basic skills of sex counselling or neglect a highly significant and important aspect of practice.

REFERENCES

1. Green, R. Taking a sexual history. In Green, R. (ed.) *Human sexuality: a health practitioner's text* (2nd edn). Baltimore: Williams & Wilkins, 1979: 22–30.
2. Reinisch, J. and Beasley, R. *The Kinsey Institute new report on sex.* New York: Penguin, 1991.
3. Laumann, E.O., Paik, A. and Rosen, R.C. Sexual dysfunctions in the United States: Prevalence and predictors. JAMA, 1999; 281: 537–544.
4. Merrill, J.M., Laux, L.F. and Thornby, J.I. Why doctors have difficulty with sex histories. *South Medical Journal,* 1990; 83: 613–617.
5. Lief, H.I. Why sex education for health practitioners? In Green, R. (ed.) *Human sexuality: a health practitioner's text* (2nd edn). Baltimore: Williams & Wilkins, 1979: 2–10.

2 *How to take a sexual history*

The sexual history should be seen as a specific application of history taking, which follows the same principles and pattern as taking a general history. It differs, however, in four respects. First, it may engender embarrassment in patient, practitioner or both. Second, it is likely, unless competently carried out and accepted by the patient, to lead to a greater proportion of false responses (usually false negatives) than any other form of medical history except possibly a psychiatric history. Third, because sexual anatomy and function are subject to circumlocutions, particular care to establish that the language used is appropriate must be taken. And fourth, because of potential embarrassment and inaccuracy in responding, it may be useful to explain the reasons for taking a sexual history, particularly when the history is not being taken in direct response to a sexual presenting problem. For these reasons, a sexual history needs to be approached with more preparation than a general history.

WHOM TO TAKE A SEXUAL HISTORY FROM?

Many authors suggest that a full sexual history should be taken from all patients. In a perfect system—where time constraints, embarrassment of practitioner and patient, and a lack of acceptance of sexuality as an integral part of physical and psychosocial functioning are not problems—this would be the approach of choice. However, because health practitioners are affected to some extent by all of the above problems, sensible utilization of time and the need to maximize the detection of problems dictate that different approaches and indices of suspicion should apply. At least five useful criteria for deciding how to approach a sexual history can be identified.

Age

Taking a sexual history for the very young is considered inappropriate unless there is reason to believe that sexual activity may have occurred. If this is the case, then the issues involved in taking sexual histories from children require an approach totally different from that used in taking a history from adults. Taking such a history requires special training and may ultimately require referral to a child psychiatrist or psychologist. Legal considerations must also be taken into account, as discussed in chapter 12. On the other hand, it is necessary for the practitioner to take sexual histories for most patients from mid-adolescence through to late adulthood. For those who are assumed to be sexually active, the issue should be raised. At the other end of the spectrum, taking a sexual history from an aged widow or widower may also be difficult because of greater embarrassment in some older people about sex, less frequent sexual activity and greater difficulty in recall.

Gender

Gender differences necessitate different approaches when taking the sexual histories of men and women. In the case of women, issues such as gynaecological functioning, contraception and parity make it easier for the practitioner to raise questions of sexuality. In men this can be more difficult, although it has been suggested that men are less reticent in discussing sexuality than women (such gender differences are probably disappearing). Double standards of sexual behavior, whereby it is more acceptable for men than women to have multiple sexual contacts or contacts outside relationships, mean it is more likely that the issue of STDs may need to be investigated in men. Conversely, such double standards may also place a female partner at risk of infection from her spouse.

Culture

Different cultures have different taboos about both sexual activity and sex-related discussions. In some cultures (e.g., Somali, Hmong), it may be necessary for the patient and health practitioner to be of the same gender in order for an accurate history to be taken. In other cultures, sexual words (e.g., 'homosexual', 'sexually active') have very different meanings. Practitioners need to know ahead of time the culture of their patients and, specifically, the language and rules for discussing sex within the culture, in order to take both a sensitive and an accurate history.

Context

The context of the consultation will also influence the sexual history. The reason for the presentation, the pressure of time, the possibility of follow-up or of taking a fuller history at a later stage, whether the consultation is single or a joint one, and the perceived confidentiality of history and records, are all factors that may determine whether a screening or a full sexual history is taken. Whether you are the regular practitioner or are seeing the patient on a one-time basis may also be a consideration. For example, in the emergency room setting a lack of privacy and lack of established relationship with the patient may affect the probability of obtaining an accurate history. In such cases, the practitioner needs to make a clinical decision about what priorities exist, in what order they should be approached, and how to best ensure that confidentiality and sensitivity are maximized.

Individual differences

The greatest barrier to taking a sexual history is sexual/moral conservatism on the part of practitioner, patient or both. Clearly, taking a sexual history from someone with conservative views will be more difficult and may yield less co-operation and/or poorer accuracy. In general, more conservative individuals are likely to have discussed sexual matters less, to have more questions about sexuality and sexual functioning, and to have greater difficulties with sexuality than more liberal individuals (though we have been consistently surprised at how wrong we have been in our judgements of patients' comfort levels with sexual issues). Thus, while practitioners may have concerns about raising the issue of sexual health with apparently conservative patients, there may be disproportionate advantages in doing so. Patients with a history of sexual abuse or for whom sexuality has in some way been emotionally painful may have greater difficulty in answering questions. In such situations, it is important that the practitioner gives herself or himself enough time to take the sexual history in a sensitive and informed way.

Similarly, conservative practitioners may be more reticent than liberal practitioners about investigating their patients' sexual lives. In our experience, such physicians may rationalize their own discomfort by arguing either that sexual history taking is not necessary or that their non-investigation will save the patient from embarrassment. Whether liberal, moderate or conservative, it is incumbent upon all practitioners, first, to be *aware* of any personal biases that may affect their patients' health; second, to develop a *plan* to ensure that personal bias does not negatively impact on the health of their patients; and third, to consistently *implement* the plan.

Despite large individual differences among practitioners and patients, which may influence either the decision to take a sexual history or the thoroughness of such a history (a few screening questions versus a full history), we advocate that all practitioners should, at a minimum, make an assessment of what the chance of sexual problems may be in their patients, and base this on information rather than guesswork.

Intellectual capacity

Intellectual handicap is a specialized field.[1] Wherever possible, close liaison with parents and involved professionals is strongly recommended.

WHEN TO TAKE A SEXUAL HISTORY?

Timing of the sexual history is important if it is to be accepted by the patient. Green[2] notes that the optimal time is not when the patient's initial visit has been prompted by influenza, nor on the third anniversary of the practitioner–patient relationship. The timing will depend on the reason why the practitioner needs to take a sexual history. Green argues that a sexual history should be taken whenever a full history is taken. However, we feel that the time to take a sexual history will depend on a number of factors, and that the most important of these is the *reason* the sexual history is taken. Three primary reasons for taking a sexual history are screening, a particular need for diagnosis and a specific sexual presenting problem.

Screening sexual history

The screening sexual history can be taken at any time and for any patient, but is recommended for patients from whom a sexual history has never been taken, or for patients who may not be receptive to having a full sexual history taken. Still, the timing is important. When a new patient is being seen, the screening questions should be asked in the context of the general history. When the patient has been seen previously, it is appropriate to add the screening questions into either relevant history, or into the preventive interview (discussed below). For both women and men, the screening questions are the same (see Box 2-1).

Screening history in women

For women, the screening history should be associated with and follow from relevant areas of the medical or psychosocial history: history of pregnancy or childbearing, history of gynaecological problems, history of STDs or other genital infections, or history of Pap smears and other investigations. Box 2-2 adds a question screening for sexual dysfunction in women.

BOX 2-1

Basic screening questions

1. When was the last time you engaged in sexual activity?
2. In the past, have you been sexual with men, women, or both?
3. With approximately how many people have you been sexual in the past year?
4. How are things going for you, sexually?
5. What questions or concerns do you have about your sexuality at this time?

BOX 2-2

Sexual functioning screening questions

1. (Female) Do you have any problems with sexual functioning; for example, problems with arousal, lubrication, pain during sexual activity, or orgasm?
2. (Male) Do you have any problems with sexual functioning; for example, problems getting aroused, or getting or maintaining an erection, or problems with ejaculation or orgasm?

Screening history in men

Much the same pattern should occur in taking a screening history for men. Again, a screening history is appropriate for patients from whom a sexual history has never been taken, or for patients who it is felt may not be receptive to having a full sexual history taken. However, opportunities for asking the screening questions are fewer in the case of men. When a new patient is being seen, the questions should be asked following the history of any urological complaints or genital infections, bowel function, or relationship problems. When the patient has been seen previously, such questions may be asked in relevant areas of history taking or in preventive history sections as discussed in chapter 8. Box 2-2 adds a question screening for sexual dysfunction in men.

Reasons for adding screening questions

In asking screening questions about sexual history, the practitioner is seeking to communicate to the patient that sexual questions are acceptable and that he or she is open to sexual problems being brought up in the consultation. This acts as a provision of permission to discuss sexual questions or problems and confirms that the practitioner can be seen as competent to answer, treat or refer on sexual issues. The investment may pay off in the future when sexual issues arise. Second, it provides an opportunity to address any existing sexual problems, or to answer immediate questions. If sexual problems are apparent, then a fuller history can be taken. Finally, it alerts the practitioner to areas of further investigation or of preventive education.

Taking a sexual history as part of a full history

Green[2] advocates that a full history should be taken on the first visit. People for whom such an approach might be appropriate will depend to some degree on the individual patient, the reason for the visit, and the confidence of the practitioner in initiating such an approach. It is worth quoting Green:

> The opening statement can be: 'As your physician, I will be responsible for helping to maintain your health in all areas... One area of health which has been relatively neglected by physicians in the past is sexual health... You should know that what we discuss is confidential, in the same way as the rest of your medical history.'
> (p. 25)

A full-frontal approach to taking a sexual history may be appropriate for patients who the practitioner believes to be relatively comfortable with issues of sexuality and who are usually younger in age. However, such a full history may not always be the approach of choice for a number of reasons, relating to the practitioner, the setting and the patient, although it is the most thorough approach for the practitioner with the time, experience and comfort to carry it out.

The general sexual history in the absence of a specific sexual complaint should cover a number of areas, including a history of how much the patient knows about sex, sexual experiences in childhood, the experience of puberty, commencement of sexual activity, sexual partners, sexual practices, current sexual relationships, history of sexual dysfunctions, history of STDs and drug history, as well as details of parity, or contraceptive or prophylactic practices as appropriate.

Taking a sexual history for specific presenting problems

For a patient presenting with a specific sexual problem such as a possible STD, a sexual dysfunction or a particular question about sexual functioning, a specific history should be taken. These problems are covered in the following chapters, because the nature of the problem will determine the approach, the questions and the issues that need to be covered to enable differential diagnoses. In this situation, the patient and the practitioner are in agreement on the need to take a sexual history. This is a natural opportunity to ask questions about sex, and thus the issues of embarrassment, inaccurate answers or dissimulation, or rationale for the history taking, are not so salient.

It is important not to overdo disclaimers. Coleman[3] suggests to students, 'You don't give lengthy explanations for other sensitive examinations; if you think it's relevant, you ask questions. If the patient is hesitant, you can always give an explanation for the line of questions. I think the main point should be that it should be part of a full history and that questions should flow easily from one part of the history to the next.'

Taking a sexual history in relation to marital or emotional difficulties

Green[2] has argued that conflicts over sexuality can result in depression, anxiety, and alcohol and other drug abuse. Lief[4] notes that more people are troubled by marital and family relationships than by any other aspect of life such as work, money, recreation, or even addictive problems related to alcohol or drugs. We know that three out of four cases of significant marital disharmony include sexual problems. Such problems are most frequently those of discrepancies in desire and perceived sexual inadequacy.

Where relationship issues or problems occur (and these may emerge only after sensitive probing by the practitioner when patients present with generalized psychosocial problems such as anxiety, depression, insomnia, tension or restlessness), questioning as to underlying sexual difficulties is essential. A general introduction followed by more specific queries is the approach of choice (see Box 2-2).

At this stage, the practitioner may move into taking a fuller sexual history as appropriate to the problem and as described in the following chapters. Alternatively, the practitioner may wish to complete a general screening of sex-related concerns. A list of other screening questions appears in Box 2-3. It is wise to have at the back of your mind the possibility that sexual

---

BOX 2-3

Other sexual questions to include in a general screen

1. What do you do to protect yourself from unplanned pregnancy?
2. What do you do to protect yourself from getting an STD or HIV? (Or for HIV positive patients: What do you do to prevent yourself from passing HIV on to others?)
3. Is there anything else that I need to know about your sexuality in order to provide you with good health care?

---

problems are commonly associated with relationship disharmony—as a cause, a symptom or a consequence—and that this possibility should always be investigated.

WHERE TO TAKE A SEXUAL HISTORY?

It would seem obvious that a sexual history should be taken in a clinical setting. However, because of the sensitivity of the issue, confidentiality should be assured. The history should not be taken with a third person present unless consent has explicitly been sought and given: having a receptionist or assistant coming in and out of a room can seriously inhibit the process. Similarly, in emergency rooms and wards where cubicles are separated by curtains and where conversations several cubicles away can be accurately overheard, sexual questioning should only be attempted if the practitioner can assure the patient of reasonable confidentiality—and taking a full sexual history should not be attempted.

The sexual history should not be commenced when the patient is in stirrups or in any other vulnerable position. When the patient is likely to feel uncomfortable or threatened, discomfort, embarrassment and dissimulation are likely to be heightened. Similarly, closeness is related to comfort. Sitting either too close or at too great a distance may convey opposite, but nevertheless potent, messages. A third issue relating to context is eye contact. Avoiding eye contact conveys embarrassment on the part of a participant. Conversely, in the context of a sexual history, seeking eye contact may seem to convey such intentions as voyeurism. It is wise to position oneself where eye contact can be both met and avoided; for example, facing, but not directly in front of, the patient.

LANGUAGE IN TAKING A SEXUAL HISTORY

A number of simple rules about language and the order of questions apply when taking a sexual history. This is perhaps the most difficult area for health practitioners once they have embarked on taking a sexual history. The difficulty is knowing whether the patient understands the medical or anatomical language used or, conversely, whether using colloquial language will offend.

Kinsey's Rule

This rule states that you should never invite a negative answer by asking people 'Have you ever . . .?'. In an area of embarrassment, most people will answer 'No' to everything but the most inescapably obvious behavior. Kinsey and colleagues[5] always phrased their questions 'When was the last time you . . .?' or 'How often do you . . .?'. This provides evidence that the practitioner is accepting of sexual variation and that no value judgements are being made. Never pose a question in such a way that a negative answer is the easiest response.

Goldman's Rule

This rule states that you should never assume that people know what words mean. Goldman and Goldman,[6] in their classic book on children's sexual thinking, provide a number of amusing examples of what people think particular anatomical and behavioral terms, in common use among health practitioners, mean. The uterus was thought to be a tunnel in Switzerland and a virgin was defined as a member of an ethnic group! Adults appear to have similar problems. It is embarrassing for one author to recollect giving a lecture on AIDS to a final-year high school class, which focussed on risk behaviors. At the conclusion of the talk, one person in the class asked what 'heterosexual' meant. On being asked, over a quarter of the class had no idea what the term, which was integral to the discussion, meant. It was assumed to be some abnormal behavior. Similarly, many patients confuse 'homosexual behavior' with 'anal intercourse'.

It is important that practitioners and patients use language that both understand. If confusion is suspected, it is helpful to have the patient describe his or her understanding of what specific words mean. Anatomical charts are also extremely useful and should be kept to hand if one is contemplating taking a sexual history. Because circumlocutions and euphemisms abound, it is not uncommon for practitioner and patient to take the same term to mean something different.

Orwell's Rule

This rule, which is related to Goldman's Rule, is named after the English novelist George Orwell, who believed that you should never use a long word when you could use a short one. The more complex or latinate the word, the more likely it is to be misunderstood. Whenever possible, ascertain what the patient's vocabulary is and use it. On the other hand, for some patients, having the practitioner use colloquial or vulgar terms may offend or give the impression that professionalism is being sacrificed. A helpful hint in starting a history is to ask the patient what kind of words he or she prefers to use in talking about sex, and to take the cue from the patient. A sensible middle approach is to describe acts ('Do you put your penis in her mouth?' rather than 'Do you engage in oral sex?'; 'Do you come?' rather than 'Do you achieve orgasm?'), where there is less confusion. In general, neutral colloquial terms are better than vulgar ones or street language, but it is essential to make sure that the terms are common in meaning. If either party is at all embarrassed, it is almost certain that confusion will be compounded.

Mitford's Rule

A cardinal rule of interviewing, described by the author Jessica Mitford (in the context of investigative journalism), is to start with the kind or easy questions, and to leave the cruel or more difficult ones until the end. In taking a sexual history, a similar principle applies. You should commence with the less confronting issues and put the patient at ease before asking more explicit and possibly embarrassing questions. This provides an opportunity for the practitioner to gain the confidence of the patient and to develop some degree of empathy. It is a mistake to commence with the most challenging or sensitive issues: they should be built up to and left to the last if at all possible.

THE ISSUE OF EMPATHY

A major problem in taking a sexual history is embarrassment (on both sides) when discussing matters that have not previously been discussed professionally. This discomfort can be overcome in two ways: through explanation and through practice.

Explanation of reasons for sexual history

Traditionally, it has been uncommon for practitioners to explain the ratio-nale for taking histories, although this is changing rapidly. It has become increasingly accepted that the patient is the practitioner's best ally in treat-ment and health maintenance. One form of explanation suggested by Green[2] has already been described above. However, a less formal approach is to tell the patient that there are a number of things you need to know in order to treat or to make a diagnosis. For example, partner numbers are a guide to assessing risk for STDs, and are necessary for contact tracing if infection is present. Sexual practices are a guide to which sites need to be investigated for STDs, and are necessary to determine whether sexual dys-functions are universal or specific to certain behaviors. Sexual contexts are a guide to whether dysfunctions may be situation-specific. Simple explana-tions both provide a rationale for the questions and give the patient some feeling of being consulted and having some control over what may be a difficult process for them. Providing a clear rationale for asking the history conveys respect, competence and concern, and thus increases the chance of accurate responses from the patient.

Practice

It is unrealistic to expect practitioners to take competent sexual histories without some practice in desensitizing discomfort. Green[2] suggests that the most eye-opening exercise for practitioners in revealing sexual-history-taking distress is a practice session or role-play. The first step is to choose a professional colleague, preferably of the same sex, to help you practise asking questions about sex. Start by asking questions about the 'patient's' sexual practices and areas of sexual conflict. In particular, listen and watch for hesitancies, vocal tone changes and facial hints in the interviewer, or signs of interviewee distress such as eye contact deflection, fidgeting or other tension. At the end of this session, have the 'patient' provide feedback on what she or he found helpful and what created discomfort. If possible, audiotape or videotape the interview to enhance the review. One approach to taking a full sexual history is outlined in Box 2-4. We recommend that practitioners use this template to practise taking a history.

The second step is to role-play a particular sexual problem, and to alter-nate the roles of patient and practitioner several times. This should be

17

BOX 2-4

Questions to ask when taking a full sexual history

I'd like to take a sexual history, and to do that, I need some general information first—then we can focus on specific areas. Is that OK?

1. For many people, it makes sense to break their sexual history up into meaningful chunks; for example, childhood and teenage years, dating and first experiences, settling down/marriage. If you were to divide your life up into three or four meaningful segments, roughly when would those be?

2. Let's then focus on the first segment (usually childhood, puberty and early adolescence).

   How much did you know about sex growing up? How did you learn? What messages about sex did you receive? Many children play 'doctors and nurses' or other games to find out about sex. What do you remember? Were you ever caught? What happened? At what age do you remember starting to masturbate? How did you learn about it? What sexual concerns did you have growing up? Anything particularly memorable? Any sexual contact with adults or children a lot older than you when you were growing up? How do you feel about this now? Anything else significant about that period?

3. Focussing on the next segment (usually adolescence, early dating and first intercourse).

   What was adolescence like for you? (Probe: In terms of sexual awakening). Were you popular or more of a loner? How old were you when your body started changing? (Probe: Did you go through puberty earlier than, at the same time as, or after your classmates?) How much did you know about these changes? Adolescence is often a time of sexual exploration for many kids. What sort of things happened for you? What concerns did you have at that time? In terms of sex, what were your goals at that time? (Probe: To wait until marriage, to get laid?) Where did these messages come from? What about same-sex experiences/sexual contact with other boys/girls? (For lesbian/gay identified patients: What about other sex experiences? Sex with women/men? How much pressure did you feel

---

to have vaginal sex? What was that like for you?) How do you feel about that now?

Let's look at the first time you had some sort of sex with someone else. Who was it with? What happened? What was it like for you? (Probe: Scary? Wonderful?) How did you feel afterwards? What happened to the relationship? After this, what was your typical sexual pattern? (Probe: Some people during this period tend to date one person; others a number; and still others, to explore with a lot of partners.) What sort of sex are we talking about? What protection did you use? Who decided that?

Looking back, what was most difficult about that period of your life? Anything else significant about that period?

4. Focussing on the next segment (usually first long-term relationship or marriage).

How old were you when you met your spouse/partner? How long after meeting did you start being sexual together? How did you decide to have sex? What was the first time like? What sort of protection did you use? Who decided that? If you look at your sex life over the relationship, what sort of patterns do you see? (Probe: For couples with children, how did having children change your sexual relationship?) How do you feel about the changes in sex over time? What was/is the best part of having sex with your partner? What have been the greatest challenges or frustrations?

For patients with no history of monogamy: What's the longest period of time you have been with only one person? Have you ever had sex with only one partner for a year or longer? (If no, probe: Why do you think this is?)

What about sex with anyone else during this period? (If yes, probe: What happened? How did you tell your partner? What protection was used?) Anything else significant about that period?

5. Focussing on the next segment (in situations of divorce, multiple relationships, widowhood).

What happened next? (Probe: How did the relationship end?) How do you feel about that now? What did/do you do

—continued overleaf

BOX 2-4 — *continued*

to take care of your sexual and intimacy needs? What has been your typical pattern since then? How do you determine when to use protection? Any particularly negative experiences or difficulties that it would be helpful for me to be aware of? Anything else significant about that period?

6. Currently, about how many male and female partners are you being sexual with? (For persons with only one partner, probe: Do you know if your partner has had sex with anyone else?) About how often are you being sexual? How satisfying is it for you? What sort of protection do you use? About how often do you use condoms? (Probe: What things determine if you use protection?) What sexual concerns or issues do you have currently? What about intimacy needs, loving and feeling loved, touch needs and being touched?

7. Ideally, how often would you like sex? What sort of sexual life would you like, ideally? In terms of oral, anal or vaginal sex, ideally what would you like? How does your current life compare with your ideal? What other sexual concerns do you have? How concerning or distressing are these?

8. We've looked at your history, some current concerns and what sort of sexual life you'd ideally like to have. Sex is an area of health where many people have concerns that they may feel shameful about or bad about. Is there anything we haven't touched on that would be important to mention, in order to best help you?

---

repeated using a colleague of the opposite sex, or a partner or spouse. Because of the sensitive nature of a sexual history, feedback is critical (far more so than in any other area of medical *or* psychological history taking) to minimize discomfort for both practitioner and patient.

Our experience is that often practitioners are more embarrassed than patients when sexual issues are raised. This is not surprising: in general, medical and other health practitioners are among the more socially conservative in the population. The interviewer who is ill at ease discussing sexuality communicates this to the patient. In turn, this can inhibit patient communication and bias patient responses.

Discomfort

Because professional people spend a longer time preparing for university admission and prioritizing their professional studies, for some the experience of sexuality in late adolescence and early adulthood may not be as extensive or may occur later than in other sectors of the population. Class differences in sexual behavior exist. People of lower socioeconomic status and those who are less educated tend to start their sexual experience earlier and have a greater variety of partners.[5,7] Conversely, the range of sexual practices is greater among the more educated and among professionals.

The consequence of these differences is that the practitioner may allow moral values to enter into the sexual-history-taking procedure, either subtly (through vocal tone or expression, or facial expression) or overtly. Our private attitudes may favor the lifestyle of one person over another. However, this attitude does not belong in the clinical interview or in responsible patient management. That is not to say that when advising on preventive aspects of sexual health, risks or consequences of particular practices should be avoided: quite the opposite. However, the practitioner's private belief about termination of pregnancy, marital monogamy, or homosexuality, for example, is irrelevant in the context of the fact-finding sexual history. Even if a practitioner's discomfort makes referral a responsible option, such a referral should be accompanied by a competent letter setting out the relevant findings and if possible a formulation of the problem.

In summary, taking a sexual history should be an integral part of the skills of health practitioners. However, it is usually not taught or is taught with severe time restrictions or minimal practice. Because of the discomfort felt by many practitioners and patients about discussing sexuality, taking a sexual history cannot (like almost any other clinical exercise) be taught solely from a book. In addition to the guidelines above, *practice* (which includes feedback from colleagues and partners) is an essential way to add sensitivity and polish to an area of history taking that requires these qualities more than almost any other area of clinical work.

REFERENCES

1. Craft, A. (ed.) *Mental handicap and sexuality: issues and perspectives.* Tunbridge Wells: Costello, 1987.
2. Green, R. Taking a sexual history. In: Green, R. (ed.) *Human sexuality: a health practitioner's text* (2nd edn). Baltimore: Williams & Wilkins, 1979: 22–30.
3. Coleman, E. Personal communication, 1999.

4. Lief, H.I. Why sex education for health practitioners? In Green, R. (ed.) *Human sexuality: a health practitioner's text* (2nd edn). Baltimore: Williams & Wilkins, 1979: 2–10.

5. Kinsey, A.C., Pomeroy, W.B. and Martin, C.E. *Sexual behavior in the human male*. Philadelphia: W.B. Saunders, 1948.

6. Goldman, R. and Goldman, J. *Children's sexual thinking*. London: Routledge and Kegan Paul, 1984.

7. Kinsey, A.C., Pomeroy, W.B., Martin, C.E. and Gebhard, P.H. *Sexual behaviour in the human female*. Philadelphia: W.B. Saunders, 1953.

3 Taking a sexual history

BEFORE YOU BEGIN

Make sure that the physical setting you provide conveys a feeling of comfort and ease. For example, where possible, softer lighting is preferable to harsh lighting, and taking the history while sitting at the desk is preferable to asking questions at the examination table. Many people find that for sexual counselling and history taking it is often best to set up two similar chairs at right angles. This arrangement prevents the confrontational eye contact you can get if there is a desk between you and the patient, and allows the patient to look away when necessary. It's also less authoritarian and less intimidating. Some furniture placed between the patient and practitioner can help to provide patients with a sense of protection, but can also serve as a barrier to sharing confidences.

PLAIN SPEAKING AND RULES FOR HISTORY TAKING

It's important to use simple words. For *body parts*, particularly with children and adolescents, some people suggest that it's a good idea to ask the patient what terms he or she uses to describe them. In general, use proper medical terms such as 'penis', 'vagina' and 'anus', and explain them with models or drawings if needed. For *behavior*, follow Goldman's and Orwell's rules (see chapter 2). Hence, terms like 'penis in your mouth', 'oral–penis sex', and 'sex with men/women' are recommended over terms like 'fellatio' and 'homosexual/heterosexual sex'. Make sure that the patient understands what you mean if you use any words that are not often encountered in everyday speech.

The definition of 'sex' is critical in taking a sexual history. In a study of undergraduate students at a major U.S. university, respondents almost all indicated that peno-vaginal intercourse would constitute 'having sex'[1]. However, only 40% considered that oral-genital contact would constitute 'having sex', while only 80% considered peno-anal intercourse to be 'having sex'. Genital touching was considered by only one in eight women and one in six men to be 'sex'. Thus, the question needs to be asked in a more specific way, for example, in terms of sexual contact, sexual arousal with another person, or asking about specific behaviors. As oral-genital, peno-vaginal and peno-anal behaviors can all transmit pathogens, specificity in questioning is essential.

It's also important to establish your own rules and to follow these consistently for every patient. In this chapter, we present two common ways of taking a history. In the previous chapter, we outlined a template for taking a complete sexual history. Some practitioners may prefer to set aside a block of time to complete this history. Because most practitioners will use natural opportunities in health care as they arise to focus on various presenting concerns, this chapter focusses on key questions to ask related to specific sexual concerns.

TAKING A SEXUAL HISTORY FROM A WOMAN

Getting started

A simple question like 'Tell me what brings you here' may be all the lead-in you need. You may well be able to keep the narrative going by using nods, an attentive listening posture and encouraging noises. Give the patient as much time as she needs to tell her story before you go on to take a formal history. Be alert for signs of embarrassment or discomfort.

Remember, in cases presenting with sexual dysfunction, the patient has already taken two major steps forward—by deciding that there is a problem and by then seeking help—but she may still feel uncertain now that she is actually in a formal consultation.

When practising getting started, think about how different types of patients would respond to your questions. For example, a common opening question used by many health practitioners is, 'Are you sexually active?'. Imagine how you would answer this question as an adolescent who engages only in solo masturbation; as a gay man who sees himself as the 'passive' partner; or as someone being sexually abused or feeling disengaged in sex. Kinsey's Rule predicts that such patients may be more inclined to simply say 'No', thus preventing the practitioner from asking any further questions.

Beginning the formal history

In any interview situation, it's a good idea to begin gathering information using non-threatening topics of conversation. Most women feel relatively relaxed talking about their menstrual history, and this is a logical chronological place to start. Box 3-1 gives you some ideas for questions. Question 6

BOX 3-1

Questions to ask about menstruation

1. How old were you when your periods started?
2. Were you prepared for the start of your periods? (Probes: Parents, schools, peers.)
3. Have you ever had any difficulties with your periods? (Probes: Premenstrual tension, irregularity, heavy bleeding, pains or cramps, other.)
4. If you are still having periods, how regular are they?
5. If you are not still having periods, can you tell me what happened before they finally stopped?
6. How did your parents express their thoughts and feelings about sex? (Probes: Expressions of affection? Attitudes to sexuality?)

BOX 3-2

Questions to ask about pregnancies

1. How many times have you been pregnant?
2. Can you tell me what happened with each pregnancy? (Probes: Medical problems, planned or unplanned pregnancy, miscarriages, terminations.)

is particularly important as it introduces the idea that the interview will be about feelings as well as facts.

Watch body language at this time. Is your patient sitting in a relaxed posture? Does her voice convey anxiety or discomfort?

Obstetric history

This may seem a little out of place, but again it's a fairly safe topic. Box 3-2 outlines some questions to use here. It's particularly important at this stage to convey a non-judgmental attitude to the woman who reveals that she has had one or more terminations. One author put her foot in it firmly when she responded to a patient's report of an abortion by saying, 'Oh, you

25

BOX 3-3

Questions to ask about intercourse history

1. Tell me what happened the first time you had sexual intercourse.
2. How did you feel about it at the time? (Probes: Worries about pregnancy, worries about sexual competence, guilt, emotional involvement with partner.)
3. What were your physical responses? (Probes: Lubrication, orgasm.)
4. Tell me about experiences after that.

---

poor thing. That must have made you feel terrible'. The patient, perhaps as a defensive rationalization, had taken the attitude that the pregnancy was a reassurance that all was well with her reproductive system and was very angry that she was being pushed into feeling guilty.

Intercourse history

By this time the woman will have picked up the idea that sexual matters are being discussed in a sensible and professional manner. Again, you need to be sensitive to verbal and non-verbal indications of tension or embarrassment. Don't make the assumption that your patient first experienced intercourse in the context of a long-term relationship, nor assume that all her sexual relationships have been heterosexual. It's probably a good idea to frame a direct question about homosexual contacts. If the answer is negative, you might go on to ask if there had ever been a situation where the woman might have wished that it had happened. Box 3-3 gives some sample questions about intercourse history.

Current sexual relationship

In this section of the history you will build up a picture of what is happening in the current relationship—how it began, what emotional and sexual factors are operating, and what the couple's power structure is like. If the patient is involved in more than one relationship, remember that her sexual and emotional responses may be quite dissimilar with regard to the different partners. Again, a non-judgmental attitude is essential. In cases of

---

BOX 3-4

Questions on her current sexual relationship

1. How did you meet your current partner? (Probes: Where? How long ago? What attracted you to him/her? Dating pattern?)
2. What happened physically in the early stages of the relationship? (Probes: How did the patient respond to kissing? cuddling? petting?)
3. What happened when you first had intercourse with your partner? (Probes: What led up to it? Situation? Who decided on intercourse? Patient's emotional response? Her sexual response? Contraception?)
4. What sort of person is your partner? (Probes: Good points? Bad points?)
5. How is the relationship going? (Probes: Good things? Bad things?)

---

sexual dysfunction at least one partner views the dysfunction as a problem. You need to find out which one and what effect it has had on them both. Box 3-4 suggests some lead-in questions.

Current sexual behaviors

This section of the history gives you a clear picture of the patient's current sexual practices. Don't be surprised that a small percentage of women will tell you that they simply don't know whether or not they have ever had an orgasm.

The section on infertility is particularly important. The mechanization of timing and positions for intercourse when couples are trying to conceive can ruin a previously happy sexual relationship (see chapter 6). Box 3-5 offers some questions.

Lesbian and bisexual women

Many lesbian and bisexual women will present to a women's health centre or a lesbian practitioner if they have the choice. Sometimes that choice is simply not available. If you have little knowledge of lesbian sexuality, we

---

BOX 3-5

Questions on current sexual behaviors

1. Currently, do you tend to have sex with men, women or both?
2. Tell me about your current sexual intercourse pattern. (Probes: Partners, emotional involvement with partners.)
3. About how often do you have intercourse? (Probes: Does this suit you? Your partner?)
4. About how often do you reach a climax when making love? If you do not climax, do you fake it? What are your reasons for that?
5. Do you have any problems with lubrication?
6. What form of contraception do you use? (Probes: Satisfaction of the method for the woman, her partner?)
7. Have you had any problems getting pregnant? (Probes: Her problem? Her partner's problem? Investigations? Interventions, pharmacological and surgical? Effects on sexual and emotional relationship?)
8. About how often do you masturbate or pleasure yourself sexually?

---

suggest you consult JoAnn Loulan's book.[2] It is not only sensible and explicit, but also has a good bibliography.

Sexual dysfunction

Sexual problems may be organic in origin, but many are psychogenic. Box 3-6 lists possible organic causes. Of course, it's essential to screen for organic factors. Even if a clear-cut organic cause is found, the sexual dysfunction is likely to have ramifications in terms of the response of the woman and her partner to the problem. Counselling may be needed, especially if the problem cannot be fixed.

Anorgasmia

This is probably women's most common complaint. They make love with a partner they care about, become sexually aroused, but do not reach a climax. The problem may be primary, where the woman has never had an orgasm, or secondary, where failure to reach orgasm develops later. (The word 'failure' is tell-tale here. Either or both partners may perceive the lack

BOX 3-6

Some possible organic causes of dysfunction

1. Acute or ongoing illness, especially if there is fever or lethargy.
2. Cardiovascular disease—there is a popular myth that sex is dangerous after infarct.
3. Endocrine disorders such as Addison's disease.
4. Diabetes—some women report loss of libido and anorgasmia.
5. Chronic illness such as arthritis, emphysema, multiple sclerosis, chronic benign pain. These are dealt with more fully in chapter 9.

of orgasm as a failure.) Make sure that the matter is not simply one of not allowing enough time. Some authorities estimate that it takes about 45 minutes for the average woman to move from initial arousal to climax other than by masturbation.

Some anorgasmic women in this situation feel sexually dissatisfied and may suffer abdominal pain resulting from vasocongestion. Another group is typified by the anorgasmic woman who responded to a question about whether she was sexually satisfied after intercourse. 'I feel great. He's the one who gets upset.' Remember that almost every woman from time to time experiences intercourse that does not lead to orgasm—what Alex Comfort[3] refers to as the 'wrong man at the wrong time' scenario. This is not anorgasmia. Some questions to ask about anorgasmia appear in Box 3-7.

General sexual dysfunction

Here the woman experiences little or no response to sexual stimulation. She does not feel aroused and the physiological responses—abdominal vasocongestion, ballooning of the vagina with the formation of the orgasmic platform, lubrication—are all absent. Sexual intercourse is likely at best to be uncomfortable and unrewarding and at worst downright distasteful.

Some women seem not to mind their unresponsiveness and here presentation is usually a result of the partner's initiative. Other women find the condition most distressing. The impact on the couple varies greatly. It is most disruptive when the woman avoids the initiation of intercourse by such means as going to bed at a different time from the partner or having the traditional 'headache'.

BOX 3-7
Questions to ask about anorgasmia

1. How do you and your partner initiate sexual intercourse? What normally happens?
2. How do you respond when she/he wants to be sexual? What happens for you?
3. What happens during foreplay? (Probes: Touching? Where? Time spent? Variety?)
4. How do you feel sexually during foreplay? (Probes: Sexual responsiveness of body parts such as nipples and vagina? Level of relaxation?)
5. Do you begin to lubricate during foreplay?
6. For vaginal and anal intercourse: how do you feel when your partner inserts his penis? (Probes: Sexually? Emotionally?)
7. How do you feel after intercourse? (Probes: Relaxation level? Sexual satisfaction? Abdominal discomfort? Emotional closeness to partner?)
8. How often do you masturbate or pleasure yourself sexually? (Probes: Climax? How long does it take you to reach orgasm? Any guilt feelings? Other feelings?)

Anxiety may be a causal or contributing factor. Assess it by direct questioning and observation of such non-verbal cues as body language and tone of voice. Anger and hostility to the partner may also be implicated.

This is an area where the woman's early experiences with sexuality are particularly important. She may well have learned her lack of response in a family that had repressive attitudes towards sexual matters. Any unpleasant or traumatic sexual experiences such as rape may also contribute.

Unlike erectile dysfunction in the male, neither anorgasmia nor general sexual dysfunction precludes intercourse. Nonetheless, the impact on both partners in the case of a sexually unenthusiastic and unpleasured woman needs to be considered. Box 3-8 contains some questions to ask in cases of general sexual dysfunction.

Vaginismus

In vaginismus, the woman experiences an involuntary spasm of the muscles in the vaginal region. This makes intercourse painful or impossible.

BOX 3-8
Some questions in generalized sexual dysfunction

1. How did your parents express affection? (Probes: To each other? To her?)
2. What did your parents teach you about sex when you were a teenager? (Probes: Readiness to discuss? General attitude to her sexuality?)
3. Where else did you find out about sex? (Probes: Peers? School? Magazines? Informational books and leaflets?)
4. Have you had any unpleasant experiences with sex? (Probes: Rape? Exhibitionism? Dyspareunia?)
5. How do you feel when you or your partner starts to make love? (Probes: Anger? Fear of failure? Resignation or indifference?)
6. How does your partner feel about your responses?
7. Is there anything in your current situation that makes sex unpleasant or difficult for you? (Probes: Partner's hygiene? Circumcision? Possible interruptions? Tiredness?)

It is difficult to assess the incidence in the population, but studies of presentations to specialist clinics suggest that it is seen in about one in ten presentations.[4,5]

In the vast majority of cases the causes are psychological. For about one in ten the problem has an organic cause and hence a physical examination is imperative.

History taking should focus strongly on the relationship, because both partners' responses may be involved in perpetuating the problem. It's also a good idea (as in most situations) to find out why the patient is presenting at this particular time. It may be that there has been a deterioration in the relationship and she feels that she has been blamed for the problems and pressurized into seeking professional help. Some possible questions are shown in Box 3-9.

Any physical examination should be carried out as gently as possible, with the realization that the patient probably has many anxieties about being touched in the vaginal area.

BOX 3-9

Questions to ask when vaginismus is a problem

1. What happens to you when your partner initiates an intercourse situation? (Probes: Arousal? Lubrication? Response of vaginal muscles? Any penetration? Her feelings?)
2. How does your partner react when your muscles go into spasm? (Probes: Frustration? Anger?)
3. Has your partner reduced the frequency of attempted intercourse?
4. Have you ever been able to have intercourse? (Probes: Partner? Situation?)
5. If you were once able to have intercourse, can you think of anything that might have caused the change?
6. What sort of things did your parents tell you about sex when you were a teenager? (Probes: Puritanical attitudes? Warnings about pregnancy?)
7. Have you had any unpleasant sexual experiences? (Probes: Rape? Childhood sexual abuse? Partner wishing uncomfortable, painful or distasteful practices? Ambivalent feelings about partner or situation?)
8. Would you like to have penetrative sex with this partner?

Finishing up

Your aim here is to make sure that the patient leaves your office feeling more relaxed and confident than she did when she arrived. Before you finish the interview, ask if there are any areas that have not been covered. Then ask if she has any questions to ask you.

The final step is to make sure, even if you have given a referral to a sex counsellor, that the door is left open for further consultations. It is very easy for a patient to feel that she has somehow done or said the wrong thing if the consultation is obviously an end to the matter as far as you are concerned. Many patients find it very difficult to talk about sexual matters and feel betrayed and abandoned if they are simply referred elsewhere with no expression of interest in the outcome.

TAKING A SEXUAL HISTORY FROM A MAN

Getting started

It's less easy to begin a sexual history with a male patient as there is no equivalent of the 'safe' female topic of menstruation. When the presenting problem is clearly a sexual difficulty, there is an obvious place to start. In other situations, for example chronic illness, it's best to start with a 'normalizing' statement. 'Your sexual functioning is just as important as, say, your stomach function. I always ask patients a little bit about how things are going sexually.'

Early sexual history

The first step is to see what kinds of attitudes and behaviors prevailed at home, school and so on. Did he feel free to discuss sexual matters with one or both parents? How did parents express affection to him? To each other? What other sources of sex education did he have? Peers? School? Magazines? Information books and leaflets?

Then, move on to his own sexuality. Again, a 'normalizing' question can help. 'Many men's first experience of their own sexuality is a wet dream. You wake up with a damp, sticky feeling on your pyjamas. Can you remember when that first started happening to you?' (If you ask whether it happened, the patient is much more likely to deny that it did.)

Masturbation is another topic that benefits from the normalization approach. 'Most men masturbate at various times in their lives.' Check that the term 'masturbation' is understood.

Then move on to early experiences of intercourse. Pay particular attention to matters of timing. Some men who have difficulties with premature ejaculation show a clear history of *learning* the behavior. Rapid sessions in situations like a parked car or the parental home put a premium on coming quickly.

Current sexual relationships

The next area to consider is the person's current sexual relationship (or relationships). Do not assume that a person's sexual partners are all of the same sex. It is imperative to ask about current same-sex sexual experiences directly, as many people are less willing to volunteer information about same-sex contacts (see chapter 13). To gain an accurate history, avoid terms like 'homosexual', 'bisexual' or 'heterosexual'; instead ask about behavior with men (or males), women (or females), or both.

Some beginning history-takers may fear that asking especially conservative patients about sex 'with men, women or both' may shock the patient, and invite doctor ridicule. Where a patient challenges any question in a history, just provide them with a suitable rationale. For example:

Doctor: Tell me, do you have sex with men, women or both?

Patient: Doctor, what are you thinking? That I'm sort of that way . . . that I'm homosexual?

Doctor: In order to help my patients, I need to get an accurate history, so I try not to make assumptions. Does that make sense?

Patient: Yeah, I guess.

Doctor: So, currently, do you tend to have sex with men, women or both?

The overall aim in this section of the history is to find out what is happening and how satisfactory it is to the people involved. Box 3-10 outlines the areas.

BOX 3-10

Questions on current sexual relationships

1. About how often do you have sexual intercourse? (Probes: How well does that suit you? Your partner(s)?)

2. Do you have any problems getting or maintaining an erection? (Probes: For how long? Partner(s)? Situation? Anxiety about it?)

3. After you insert your penis, about how long does it take before you ejaculate? (Probes: Satisfaction to self? Satisfaction to partner?)

4. How enjoyable do you think your partner finds sexual intercourse? (Probes: Enjoyment of foreplay? Orgasm?)

5. About how often do you masturbate, currently?

6. What form of contraception do you currently use?

7. What sort of person is your partner? (Probes: Dominance in the relationship? Enjoyment of physical affection?)

8. If the two of you are having any sexual difficulties, how do you respond? (Probes: Own response? Partner's response? Recriminations?)

9. Have you had sex with women, men or both? (Probes: How many? Satisfaction? Emotional responses?)

Sexual dysfunction

The most common male problems are low sexual desire, erectile dysfunction, premature ejaculation and, rather more rarely, retarded ejaculation. There is a greater pressure on males than on females to perform sexually. A woman may fake an orgasm, but a man cannot fake an erection. Not only are male difficulties more obvious and more likely to make penetrative intercourse impossible, but there is a greater social expectation of male sexual competence. As we said earlier, female anorgasmia may be perceived as a failure on the part of her male partner.

When intercourse difficulties clearly relate to a man's problems, he may have feelings of inferiority, guilt and inadequacy. His partner may respond with belittling comments, anger, feelings of being sexually unattractive, and so on.

Erectile dysfunction

The plain truth of the matter is that most men will fizz once or more in their sexual lives. Problems arise when the man feels traumatized by the event and worries about a recurrence. Anxiety and tension make it less likely that he will get a functional erection.

The distinction between primary erectile dysfunction (the man has never achieved an erection sufficient for penetration) and secondary dysfunction (where the difficulty arises after previously adequate erectile capacity, or is situationally specific), is helpful in identifying onset and causes of sexual dysfunction. The main differential diagnosis that needs to be made is between organically based and psychogenic dysfunction. Problems related to medication, disease processes such as diabetic neuropathy, neurological damage, and so on need to be screened out. Even if a clear organic cause is found, most patients and their partners may have experienced significant psychological discomfort and developed unhelpful patterns (e.g., avoidance). Hence, counselling can be helpful even in cases of organic causes.

There is a double-edged sword here. Of course, no physician would want to miss an organic diagnosis. On the other hand, both the patient and his partner may have a vested interest in finding an organic cause. The patient can then say that it is not his fault. The partner need not feel that he or she is a sexually unattractive package. Sometimes, overassiduous searching for underlying pathology may encourage the belief that nothing can be done.

BOX 3-11

Questions to ask in erectile dysfunction

1. Do you ever get erections? (Probes: During the night? When you wake up? When masturbating? With erotic magazines, pictures, videos, etc.? Any exceptions?)
2. Describe what happens when you attempt to be sexual/start to make love? (Probes: Who initiates it? How? Anxiety? Anger? Fantasies?)
3. Do you begin to get an erection at all? What happens to it? (Probes: Before intercourse? Beginning intercourse? During?)
4. Is your penis getting enough physical stimulation during intercourse? (Probes: Does your penis feel numb or more sensitive? Specific to condom use?)
5. Does the problem apply to all your sexual partners? (Probes: With women/men? Workers in the sex industry? Extramarital relationships?)
6. Are you on any medications? Do you smoke?
7. How often do you drink alcohol before sexual intercourse? Do you think it affects your erections or enjoyment?
8. Do you suffer from any long-term illness? (See chapter 9 for some chronic illnesses that may affect sexual function.)
9. How does your partner react?

The questions in Box 3-11 will help you establish whether or not the dysfunction is psychogenic. If a man can get a satisfactory erection in some circumstances (say, with one partner rather than another, or during sleep) the dysfunction may reasonably be viewed as a psychological problem and be treated by behavioral methods (see chapter 6).

Premature ejaculation

There are different definitions of premature ejaculation—from the amount of time elapsed between intromission and orgasm, or the number of thrusts before the man comes, to Masters and Johnson's[6] operational definition of sufficient time after intromission for a female partner to reach orgasm on 50% of occasions. The last suggestion seems to disregard the fact that many women are anorgasmic with intercourse alone, and appears to regard premature ejaculation as an exclusively heterosexual problem.

BOX 3-12

Questions to ask in premature ejaculation

1. Can you tell me about your early experiences of masturbation? (Probes: Secrecy? Need for speed? Emotional responses?)
2. Now, think back to your early experiences with sex—what were they like? (Probes: Partners? Situations? Emotional responses? Need for rapid ejaculation? Sex industry workers?)
3. About how long do you spend in foreplay? Do you ever have to ask your partner to stop touching your penis because you are nearing ejaculation?
4. About how long does it take from the time you insert your penis to the time you ejaculate? (Probes: Satisfaction to self? Satisfaction to partner?)
5. About how long would you like to last before ejaculation? (Probe: Would your partner tend to reach orgasm in that time?)
6. Is there any way your partner can reach orgasm after you have ejaculated?
7. Has this pattern of relatively early ejaculation always been true of you? (Probes: Other partners? Homosexual contacts?)

Perhaps the most useful working definition is that the man (and/or his partner) wishes he could last longer. The most helpful knowledge to be armed with is the Kinsey Report[7] finding that about three quarters of the men sampled reported ejaculating within two minutes of intromission. At the level of providing limited information (see chapter 6), you can reassure a patient with premature ejaculation concerns by normalizing his experience.

Nonetheless, many men and their partners would like some help in prolonging intercourse time. Box 3-12 gives guidelines for interviewing and chapter 6 outlines therapeutic approaches.

Retarded ejaculation

Retarded ejaculation is when a man either takes a very prolonged period of time from intromission to ejaculation or fails to ejaculate at all. The cause may be organic, the result of medication, or psychological.

BOX 3-13

Questions to ask in retarded ejaculation

1. When you are able to come, about how long does it usually take you to come after you have inserted your penis?
2. How often do you find yourself not coming during intercourse? (Probes: With all partners? Is there any kind of situation that makes it worse? What's the usual pattern?)
3. Has this always been true of you? If not, can you think of anything that might have made things change? (Probes: Drug use? Traumatic sexual experience? Partner change?)
4. Are there any circumstances when you do ejaculate? (Probes: Masturbation? Oral sex? Anal sex? Other partners? Male partners? Sex aids? Fantasies? Condom use?)
5. How does your partner react when you take a long time to come?
6. Let's go back in time to your early experiences of intercourse. How were things then? (Probes: Partners? Situations? Any problems?)
7. Can you remember any sexual experiences that were upsetting or embarrassing to you? (Probes: Erectile dysfunction? Unwilling partner? Rape?)
8. Are you on any medications?
9. Have you had any surgery on or near your sex organs? (Probes: Penis? Testicles? Bladder? Prostate?)

Antidepressives, antipsychotics, narcotics and the benzodiazepines are among the many drugs that may cause retarded ejaculation in some patients. Often the man will notice a connection between his medication and retarded ejaculation, do a cost-benefit analysis, and perhaps take himself off the drug. Thus when treating patients with these drugs it is important to discuss and monitor sexual side effects, patient satisfaction, and their effects on patient medication compliance.

Organic causes of retarded ejaculation include diabetic neuropathy, multiple sclerosis, prostate surgery, and neurological damage. The characteristic feature of organically based retarded ejaculation is that the problem is seen in all sexual circumstances. Careful, specific questioning is needed to establish this fact.

Psychogenic retarded ejaculation can also have a variety of causes. Insufficient penile stimulation, sexual guilt, a traumatizing sexual experience, and unappealing characteristics of a particular sexual partner or relationship are the most common causes. A complete history of past and current sexual experiences may furnish clues here.

While some partners of men who show retarded ejaculation may initially be delighted by their discovery of a sexual athlete, they tend rapidly to find the phenomenon rather dull and, given a man who feels he must go on until he ejaculates, even painful.

Some men with retarded ejaculation fake orgasm to avoid the embarrassment of admitting their problem. Retarded ejaculation should always be considered a possibility when investigating infertility. Box 3-13 outlines some areas to cover.

Dyspareunia

Penile pain in intercourse almost always has an organic cause, such as urethral infection or urethral scar tissue resulting from gonorrhea or a tight foreskin. For older men, Peyronie's disease (the development of scar tissue around the sheath surrounding the spongy, penile tissues which become engorged in erection) may be a source of pain during intercourse. These causes can usually be treated directly (see chapter 15).

For a more detailed analysis of physical and psychosocial causes of dysfunction in both males and females, see Lechtenberg and Ohl.[8]

REFERENCES

1. Sanders, S.A. and Reinisch, J.M. Would you say you 'had sex' if . . . ? JAMA, 1999; 281: 275–277.
2. Loulan, J. *Lesbian sex.* San Francisco: spinsters/aunt lute, 1984.
3. Comfort, A. *The joy of sex. A gourmet guide.* London: Mitchell Beazley, 1987.
4. Bancroft, J. and Coles, L. Three years' experience in a sexual problems clinic. *British Medical Journal,* 1976: 1575–1577.
5. Meares, E. An assessment of the work of 26 doctors trained by the Institute of Psychosexual Medicine. *Public Health,* 1978; 92: 218–223.
6. Masters, W.H. and Johnson, V.E. *Human sexual inadequacy.* Boston: Little, Brown and Co., 1970.
7. Kinsey, A.C., Pomeroy, W.B., Martin, C.E. and Gebhard, P.H. *Sexual behavior in the human female.* Philadelphia: W.B. Saunders, 1953.
8. Lechtenberg, R. and Ohl, D.A. *Sexual dysfunction. Neurologie, urologie and gynaecological aspects.* Philadelphia: Lea and Febinger, 1994.

4 Sexual history taking for sexually transmissible diseases

In the last decade, the general population has become more knowledgeable about sexually transmissible diseases (STDs). With the publicity given to HIV/AIDS (and to a lesser extent, herpes), and media coverage of emerging treatments, many patients now are more aware about STDs.

Despite this, there are still a number of persistent myths about STDs, and the practitioner may need to provide basic patient education as well as a diagnosis. In particular, many people do not understand that infection may (and commonly does) occur without signs or symptoms. Some people fear that notification of diseases may lead to public exposure. Such patients may be more reluctant to answer specific sexual questions truthfully. In taking a history for STDs, more than for any other area of sexuality, it may be important to explain the reasons for particular questions.

Generally, the patient with a suspected STD presents with some suspicion of what the problem may be. On the other hand, there are a number of genital infections that are not (or are not necessarily) sexually transmitted. A word on terminology is important here. Sexually *transmissible* diseases (e.g., herpes, syphilis, HIV, hepatitis B and C) can be transmitted by sexual contact, but also by other means. Sexually *transmitted* diseases are invariably transmitted by sexual contact (e.g., gonorrhea, genital warts). The distinction is important in both taking a history and explaining to the patient the need for the history or for identifying the possible source of infection.

COMMENCING THE HISTORY

It is important to put the patient at ease, and this should be done as much as possible while taking the demographic details and history of signs and symptoms. At the same time, a thorough history of recent medication, particularly antibiotics, should also be taken—first, because antibiotics may mask the symptoms of any infection, and second, because fixed drug reactions or other effects of medications may mimic the signs of STD infections.

PREVIOUS STDS

A history of previous STD infections needs to be taken. If previous STDs have occurred, were these self-diagnosed and treated; was a presumptive diagnosis made and treatment given by a health practitioner; was the diagnosis made and confirmed by laboratory evidence? While this may seem self-evident, it is not uncommon to find that STDs were not definitively diagnosed, and thus the degree of confidence you can have in previous diagnoses is lower. If treatment occurred, it is also useful to determine whether the full course of treatment was followed. A history of STDs, together with any current exposure risk, should be a sign to the practitioner that this patient is at increased risk for HIV and other STDs. Knowing this, you should take extra time and effort in providing preventive education. Box 4-1 outlines questions to ask when taking a history of STDs.

CONFIDENTIALITY AND THE LAW

In many jurisdictions, specific STDs must be reported to the government health authorities. This is necessary for epidemiologists to monitor the incidence of STD infections and their trends over time. Also, the government may need such information to carry out contact tracing and partner notification.

The purpose of notification is frequently misunderstood by patients, who do not understand the purposes of mandatory reporting and who may fear exposure. We find it is most useful to actually show patients the notification forms if they are in any doubt, and to assure them that this information is completely confidential and will only be seen by the health practitioner and by the epidemiologist in the government health department.

In a small community, confidentiality is often of even greater concern. There have been sufficient situations with HIV infection, particularly in the early days of the epidemic, where the names of infected people have been made public either in the media or through gossip, with highly distressing and discriminatory results. Absolute confidentiality must be assured and provided, and this fact must be made clear to all those working in a practice or clinic (from medical to cleaning staff), regardless of their role. It only takes one case of breach of confidentiality to ruin a practitioner's reputation and the reputation of the clinic or practice; it is in addition unethical and could lead to professional censure or withdrawal of a licence to practise. Hence it is important to explicitly discuss confidentiality with all staff. If necessary, it can be helpful to directly discuss this concern with

41

BOX 4-1

Questions to ask when taking a history of STDs

Because STDs may be asymptomatic, it can be difficult or impossible to get a complete history. Helpful questions to ask include the following:

1. How often in the past have you had an STD check-up?
2. To the best of your knowledge, what sexually transmissible diseases have you had? (Focus on naming one disease at a time. Probes: Roughly when was this? About how many times have you had a recurrence? What sort of treatment, if any, did you get for this? How long did you wait for treatment? What did the doctor/nurse call it? What sort of education did you receive? How much do you know about this now?)
3. What about other symptoms you might have had for which you did not get treatment? (Probe: Depending on what the person has already revealed, check out specific symptoms; e.g., Have you ever noticed small blisters on your penis? What about a burning sensation when you urinate?)
4. To the best of your memory, have any of your partners, current or past, had STDs?
5. (For viral STDs) About how often do you experience an outbreak? What brings it on? How painful is it? What do you do to treat it?

---

patients, including (in small community settings) asking patients which staff they know, and what specific confidentiality concerns they have. These issues are discussed further in chapter 12, which deals with legal and ethical aspects.

HOW FAR BACK TO TAKE A HISTORY?

The short answer to this question is that a history should be taken as far back as necessary to ascertain risk of exposure, or to the point where the history becomes too uncertain to be reliable. This may vary from a total history for the individual with few sex contacts, to a history dating from before the last examination (for those who have regular STD checks), to a history of the past week for workers in the sex industry. A second criterion is to consider the incubation period of the suspected disease, and to take a history covering the longest possible incubation period plus a week. This has, however, a number of limitations.

The major limitation is that where a person is at risk for one STD, they will be at risk for others. It is a well-established fact that a significant proportion of patients presenting with STDs may have multiple infections, some of which may be subclinical. If an STD is found or suspected, it is important to check for other STDs at the same time.

A further limitation is that because many STDs will be subclinical, or 'silent' infections, there is no certainty when the infection occurred. Further, the infection may be clinically intermittent, as in the case of genital herpes. Thus, the patient may have been infected, and been infecting other people, for a long time. Even with clinical signs of an STD infection, infection may have occurred some time previously and have become clinically obvious only because of illness, alteration in immune function, or stress.

A third problem is that some infections, such as HIV or herpes, may have a long incubation time (in the case of HIV, over ten years). Thus it is difficult in some cases to take a full history over this time period, particularly where the person has had a number of sexual partners. A clinical judgment needs to be made in each case as to what method will provide the most detailed history: one that will garner the information necessary to notify contacts and determine what tests to carry out, and where.

History of numbers of sexual partners

The easiest way to take a history of numbers of sexual partners is to obtain estimates: first of lifetime sexual partners; then of partners over the past year; and then (if this is still a considerable number) of those within the maximum incubation period of the suspected STD (if one or more STDs are suspected).

Once this has been done, the history of partners should be taken working backwards, with the most recent first. We find it is helpful to ask the first names only of the partners (if known), or other details to identify them, and their gender.

The issue of partner gender is one on which many STD histories founder. Medical history taking is analogous to dancing, where the patient most frequently takes her or his cues from the practitioner. To avoid inaccurate assumptions, we refer to 'partner(s)' (genderless) and only later, after the history has commenced, do we ask about the gender if this is still unclear. The patient will almost invariably fill in the gaps by referring to the partner as '*he*' or '*she*', thus obviating the need for a direct question! A common mistake is to assume that for a female, her partner(s) will be male, and for a male that the partner(s) will be female. Where the practitioner makes this mistake (e.g., by asking a woman, 'How many men have you had sex with?' or 'What was his first name?'), he or she precludes taking a history of homosexual or bisexual contacts. A leading question that assumes that all contacts are heterosexual (or for an identified lesbian or gay person, homosexual) will in most cases elicit a substantially false history. This is probably the single most common mistake to occur in taking a sexual history in the context of STDs. Ross[1] found that between 20% and 53% of men with homosexual contacts did not admit to this fact in STD clinics (with more not admitting to such contact in countries and cultures where homosexual behavior is more stigmatized). It is important to make it clear that you are interested in sexual partners of both genders and to explicitly ask, after requesting an estimate of numbers of previous partners, whether these partners were men, women or both genders. Box 4-2 lists questions to ask when taking a history of sexual partners.

History of sexual practices

Once the numbers of sexual partners has been established, it is useful to write down the first name or initial of each partner and then go back and fill in the details of the sexual encounter. Because the details of sexual practices are necessary to make an assessment of what sites to investigate for infection, you should first ask what sexual contacts occurred (this should

---

BOX 4-2
Questions to ask when taking a history of sexual partners

1. Over your lifetime, about how many women and men (males and females) have you had sex with?
2. Currently, say in the last year, how many male and female partners have you had sexual contact with? (For persons with only one partner, probe: Do you know if your partner has had sex with anyone else?)

include contacts without ejaculation). Then for each contact, it should be established whether the following sexual activities occurred.

Vaginal intercourse

Was there any vaginal penetration by penis, by fingers or by sex toys such as vibrators or other objects? This latter point is important to assess if vaginal trauma exists or may have occurred. If vaginal sex occurred, vaginal investigations should occur.

Anal intercourse

Was there any anal penetration (this must be asked of both male and female patients)? Approximately 10–20% of heterosexual women, 20–30% of heterosexual men, and 60–75% of homosexual men have experienced some kind of anal stimulation or penetration during sex. Hence, asking about anal sex is important, as it appears to be more common than most practitioners think. If there is any suggestion of anal intercourse, then anal investigation should occur.

Oral sex

Oral sex is one of the most common practices in both homosexual[2] and heterosexual sex. It is necessary to establish, first, if oral sex occurred, and second, if it did, who inserted what into whom. The most common practices are likely to be oro-penile sex (fellatio) and oro-vulval sex (cunnilingus). However, oro-anal sex (rimming) is becoming more common in heterosexual contacts, and should be routinely asked about in cases of homosexual contacts.

Where oro-penile sex has occurred, the urethra and pharynx would be considered for culture. Where oro-vulval and oro-anal sex has occurred, urethral and vaginal, and urethral and anal, sites respectively should be investigated.

Manual sex and non-penetrative practices

Manual sex (masturbation either solo or mutual) is common and may for some people be the preferred form of sexual release. Mutual or non-shared masturbation does not in general pose a risk of STD infection. Nor does frottage (where full body contact may be used to achieve stimulation or orgasm). However, where patients feel guilty, shameful or uncertain about these activities or some aspect of the encounter, they may present seeking STD testing. Asking what was most distressing for the patient can be helpful in uncovering the specific patient concern(s). Then, providing reassurance, education and sometimes referral for counselling can be helpful—dependent on the patient's presenting concern, age, experience, knowledge and distress.

Other penetrative practices

These are less common than the above, and include use of sex toys which may possibly transmit pathogens, and brachioproctic (fisting) practices, which can occur in both homosexual (male–male and female–female) and heterosexual contexts. While it is difficult to transmit STDs this way provided there are no tears in the epithelia, HIV transmission through brachioproctic sex has been reported by Donovan and colleagues.[3] These practices are reported for the sake of completeness but it is recognized that they will figure in the more specialized practices and not form part of the sexual history in the usual course of events. Where penetrative practices may lead to trauma, STD transmission may be enhanced, and if trauma is suspected it should be investigated during the physical investigation.

Just as it is important not to make assumptions about the gender of a patient's sexual partners, it is also important not to make assumptions about sexual activities. The most common mistake here is to ask what a person 'likes to do sexually' as opposed to what they actually do. We find it is helpful to preface the history of sexual practices by a comment such as 'I am going to ask you about a range of sexual practices which we commonly have reported to us'. This will usually put the patient more at ease and make it less difficult or embarrassing to report on practices that they may feel ashamed about. One can then ask about vaginal intercourse and anal intercourse (clarifying as necessary 'receptive, insertive or both'). For oral intercourse, the terms 'receptive' and 'insertive' can be confusing. In such cases, asking about 'performing oral sex on . . .', (or 'sucking/licking') and 'being sucked' is necessary to avoid confusion. Finally, if you question the patient about a list of activities, it is prudent to finish by asking, 'Are there any other sexual activities or concerns that you have that I should know about?'. This creates an opportunity for the patient to address any historical or current concerns that may have been missed.

Condom use and contraception

Following on from the history of sexual practices, or at the same time if it is easier, the clinician should ascertain whether and how often condoms were used. It is important not to assume that condom use implies protection. If the condom was put on at the last minute, infection still may have occurred as ejaculation is not a necessary condition for STD infection.

BOX 4-3

Questions to ask when taking a risk assessment

1. About how often do you use protection when having sex with someone? How do you decide when to use protection and when not to? What do you think about that as a way of making decisions?
2. When are you most able to insist on using a condom? Reasons? When are you most at risk of not using a condom? Reasons?
3. Regardless of whether your tests come back positive or negative, what needs to happen for you to protect yourself and others in the future? (Probe: How does this address your risk situations?)

Further, inappropriate or inadequate fitting of the condom as well as breakage may also lead to infection. This possibility should be explored. Where a patient indicates less than 100% condom use, it can be very helpful to ask the patient to identify when and why a condom is or is not used, as this can assist patient education and future risk reduction. Two ways to investigate further are presented. Box 4-3 contains sample questions to ask when taking a risk assessment. Box 4-4 contains written survey questions that the practitioner can hand to the patient, and later review.

Many patients still confuse contraception and STD prophylaxis. In some patients, there may be the belief that contraceptives alone (particularly douche, spermicide or barrier methods such as the diaphragm) are sufficient protection against infection. Alternatively, where an IUD is fitted, particularly those (no longer commonly used) with a filamentous tail, infection of the pelvis should be considered and an appropriate history taken or examination performed.

Adherence

While taking a sexual history, it is also useful to form an opinion as to whether the patient is likely to adhere to treatment regimens. This can be ascertained through previous histories of compliance with medication or by determining whether the patient's social situation is likely to impose any barriers to treatment.

BOX 4-4

Reasons for unsafe sex

Think back to the last few times you did NOT use a condom in vaginal or anal sex. Why did this occur? (Check as many as apply.)

—a. I was drunk or high
—b. I was feeling depressed/just didn't care
—c. I felt so lonely
—d. I felt I really had to have sex
—e. I was with my primary partner
—f. I was with a casual partner/date
—g. I was in an anonymous situation
—h. I didn't feel I could insist
—i. I felt so much in love
—j. I was with a really hot, sexy, partner
—k. I really wanted to fuck/be fucked
—l. My partner really wanted to fuck/be fucked
—m. I did not want to use a condom
—n. My partner did not want to use a condom
—o. My partner looked like s/he had HIV/AIDS
—p. My partner looked like s/he was not infected
—q. My partner said s/he has HIV/AIDS
—r. My partner said s/he does *not* have HIV/AIDS
—s. I was with a male partner
—t. I was with a female partner
—u. Neither of us had condoms with us
—v. Never. I have never had anal or vaginal sex
—w. Never. I have never used a condom
—x. Always. I always use a condom for vaginal and/or anal sex
—y. Other (please specify):

_____

From: Rosser et al. (1999). *Evaluation of Reasons for Unsafe Sex.*[4]

PARTNER NOTIFICATION

Partner notification (also known as contact tracing) is frequently a source of concern to the patient and an obligation (in some places a legal one) of the practitioner. However, research has suggested that the most accurate partner notification is done by the patient.[5] If the patient does not want a particular partner to be notified, he or she will withhold information that will make such notification impossible. At times, there will simply not be enough information available to identify the partner (e.g., 'He was about my height and left-handed. We met behind the City Tavern').

Patients need to be given the option, where partners are identifiable, either to make the notification themselves, or to have the practitioner do it for them (anonymously if preferred). In some cases, patients will have real fears of retribution or discrimination where their identity is made known to the contact, and the practitioner should respect such concerns.

In such cases, if the patient chooses not to notify the contact personally, the practitioner can send out a form letter stating that 'We believe you may have been exposed to an infectious disease through contact with a carrier. Please contact [the clinic or practitioner] quoting the number above so that we can arrange to investigate any possible infections and treat them where appropriate'. Alternatively, many STD clinics have specialized facilities for contact tracing and may be happy to have any contacts referred on to them. This may have the additional advantage of preserving anonymity if it is possible for the contact to identify the patient from the clinic or practitioner she or he attended.

In general, if patients are willing to have partners notified, it is far more efficient and cost-effective to have them do it themselves (cards or letters may be given to them for this purpose). If patients are unwilling to have contacts notified, they will simply not co-operate, and attempting to force them to do so is counterproductive. (It destroys the physician–patient relationship, leaves patients feeling alienated, and increases lack of compliance and avoidance of attendance for future screening or symptoms).

CONCLUDING THE INTERVIEW

At the conclusion of the history, it is important to debrief the client from what may have been an embarrassing or difficult interview. This debriefing should commence with a summary (in appropriate language) of what steps are likely to be taken next in terms of investigations or treatment.

Following this, it is also important to give the patient a chance to add anything (we are all familiar with the patient who brings up a major issue in the last minutes of a consultation). Sometimes patients will want to correct information, or to make an admission that they were not entirely forthcoming once they have ascertained that the practitioner is accepting and does not make moral judgments. Clinicians who work full time in STD

49

practices are familiar with such occasions ('Actually, I did have sex with another man once . . .').

Taking time for questions at the end of the history provides the patient with an opportunity to ask questions and to receive answers that may be able to correct fears or misapprehensions, such as whether their behavior is 'normal', or what the effects of STDs may be on fertility, or what the signs and symptoms of particular STDs may be. It is important to allow these questions both from the point of debriefing and clarification, and also from the point of leading into preventive education (described in chapter 8).

Patient education is important here. The patient needs to know what STD he or she has, how it was acquired, what he or she can do to avoid transmitting the infection and what can be done to avoid further infection. Holmes et al.[6] provide a rather technical but highly informative source of background.

In summary, the STD history is designed to give the practitioner the information needed to carry out appropriate investigations, make an appropriate diagnosis, and carry out appropriate partner and epidemiological notification. It can also prepare the groundwork for preventive education. As with all sexual histories, the key to success is to take a non-judgmental attitude, explain to the patient why you are asking particular questions, and be clear why you need to ask particular questions and where they may lead you in terms of their clinical implications. Even if the decision is to refer the patient on, it will be a great help to the practitioner you refer on to if you have obtained a clear and concise history and possible differential diagnoses from which to start.

REFERENCES

1. Ross, M.W. Psychosocial factors in admitting to homosexuality in sexually transmitted disease clinics. *Journal of Sexually Transmitted Diseases*, 1985; 12: 83–86.

2. Ross, M.W. *Psychovenereology.* New York: Praeger, 1986.

3. Donovan, B., Tindall, B.D. and Cooper, D.A. Brachioproctic eroticism and transmission of the AIDS retrovirus. *Genitourinary Medicine*, 1986; 62: 390–392.

4. Rosser et al. Evaluation of reasons for unsafe sex. Man-to-Man: Sexual Health Seminars Manual. Minneapolis, MN: Program in Human Sexuality, 1999.

5. Rothenberg, R.B. and Potterat, J.J. Strategies for management of sexual partners. In Holmes, K.K., Mårdh, P.A., Sparling, P.F. and Wiesner, P.J. (eds) *Sexually transmitted diseases.* (2nd edn). New York: McGraw-Hill, 1990: 1081–1086.

6. Holmes, K.K., Mårdh, P.A., Sparling, P.F. and Wiesner, P.J. (eds) *Sexually transmitted diseases.* (2nd edn). New York: McGraw-Hill.

5 *Sexual counselling*

Modern counselling is a situation where a therapist and client together explore and delineate the client's problem, set attainable goals for therapy and devise strategies to reach those goals.

Counselling theory and practice has several main sources, including the work of Carl Rogers[1,2] and modern learning theory.

Let's begin with Rogers. He believes that human beings have an innate potential for positive change. He called it self-actualization. The role of the helping professional is simply to provide the client with a situation where growth can occur.

Rogers saw three essential ingredients that any therapist needs to provide.[3]

- Respect and unconditional positive regard for the client. While we may not always approve of everything the client does or says, we need to convey the fact that we believe he or she is basically a decent human being with the capacity to develop and grow.
- Empathic understanding. This is the willingness to listen carefully to the client, see things from his or her point of view and to communicate this understanding.
- Genuineness (congruence). This is the therapist's feeling of being comfortable with himself or herself and being able to respond spontaneously.

The implication of this approach is that the counsellor is a facilitator, who helps the patient to generate his or her own goals and strategies.

Rogers's greatest contribution to counselling is his emphasis on process. When we look at content, especially for sexual counselling, a behavioral approach is seen to be most productive.

The behavioral approach sprang from learning theory and has several characteristics:

- Much of human behavior is learned.
- Maladaptive behavior can be unlearned or more positive behaviors substituted.
- Although maladaptive behaviors were learned in the person's past, therapy focusses on the learning of new behaviors in the here and now.

In terms of sexual counselling, that means we can focus on a specific problem and treat that rather than become involved in attempts to promote major personality change.

In addition to these facets of general counselling, the sexual counsellor has a major role as an educator. In spite of the vast amounts of sexual information available in books, magazines, school programs and so on, much of the population remains in what Packard[4] called 'The Sexual Wilderness', surrounded by rapid changes in attitudes and values, myths and misinformation.

This implies that it is a paramount responsibility of the sex counsellor to be well informed—and to be willing to say, 'I don't know but I'll try to find out', when a question outside your knowledge base turns up.

Useful, practical books to enhance your counselling skills include Egan[5] and Nelson-Jones.[6]

COUPLES THERAPY

If at all possible, see both members of a partnership together. This may need a little tact to arrange, especially if one member believes it is the other person's problem. Nonetheless, any sexual difficulty will impact on a relationship and a partner's response to problems may play a part in maintaining and increasing the dysfunction.

Some therapies involve a major commitment of the partner to the treatment program (see chapter 6). Here it is essential to see the partner to maintain motivation, defuse problems and monitor progress.

The commonest scenario in sex counselling is that the patient presents alone. When the history has been taken, point out to the patient that you have been asking about the partner's response a lot of the time. The vast majority of sexual problems are experienced as relationship problems. For this reason and because of the possible involvement of him or her in treatment, you would like to talk to the partner. Reassure the patient that everything that has already been discussed by the two of you will remain confidential (see chapter 12).

It's a good idea to seek the patient's permission to telephone the partner and arrange an appointment. There are two good reasons for this. Firstly, it puts a degree of professional 'clout' behind the request. A partner is more likely to refuse to attend if the issue is broached by the original patient. Secondly, it goes some way towards defusing the idea that the therapist and the presenting patient are in an alliance against the partner.

Take a sexual history from the partner in an individual session. When you see the couple together, make it clear that they are to have equal air space. 'I'm going to ask you, X, to describe things as you see them. Then I'll ask you, Y, to tell me how they affect you.'

Even if a partner refuses to attend your rooms, it is unusual to find a person who is unwilling to take part in even a brief telephone interview.

THERAPIST SKILLS

The main points of importance are that the therapist be comfortable in the counselling situation and knowledgeable about sexuality. The skills of active listening, rapport-building and accurate empathy are central, too.

Some of these skills are common to all counselling situations, some more specific to sexual counselling.

Comfort

It is very unproductive for a practitioner to be obviously uncomfortable and evasive when discussing sexual matters. Even if you personally would prefer not to include sexuality in your work with patients, you will undoubtedly find situations where the patients themselves raise sexual matters.

Box 5-1 gives an example of a practitioner who was evasive in the face of a relatively simple question from a patient.

It's a good idea to desensitize yourself to any embarrassment you feel by doing practice interviews and role plays with colleagues and friends.

BOX 5-1
An uncomfortable practitioner

After repeated dilation and curettage had failed to reduce excessive menstrual bleeding, her gynaecologist recommended that Mrs C. have a hysterectomy. She went home, discussed the matter with her husband and returned with a series of questions. One of these was, 'Will sex still be as good with me on top?'.

She described the gynaecologist's response. 'He nearly fell off his chair, muttered that he didn't know and started asking a heap of questions about other things. He might at least have offered to try and find out.'

Knowledge

As we have said before, it is the responsibility of the practitioner to know as much as possible about the area. Most medical libraries have several texts on sexual problems (many shelved at Dewey number 616.8583).

Papers on sexual matters can be found in journals of psychiatry, psychology, gynaecology, urology and general medicine. For a broad view of sexual attitudes and behaviors in western culture, see Johnson et al.[7] and Janus and Janus.[8]

There are innumerable sex manuals in the popular press. Read as much as possible.

Rapport-building

The client needs to feel comfortable before he or she will feel able to discuss sexual matters frankly. The major ingredient here is a calm, professional approach. Feeling comfortable about your own sexuality and that of others is essential.

The physical set-up of your rooms can facilitate communication. For sexual interviews, it's a good idea to seat yourself and the patient in similar-sized chairs set at right angles. This reduces formality, is less confrontational and allows the patient to avoid eye contact with you from time to time if he or she wishes.

Two essential ingredients of rapport-building are active listening and accurate empathy.

Active listening

You can communicate the fact that you are listening carefully and actively trying to understand what you hear by both non-verbal and verbal means.

Body language is very important in conveying that we are attending closely to what a person is saying. Egan suggests five behaviors that you can adopt to signify a listening attitude (see Box 5-2).

The verbal behaviors that indicate active listening include such things as the occasional 'yes' or 'um', prompting the patient to continue talking. Do not be too afraid of silences. If you lean towards the patient and look expectant, the chances are that the story will continue. Silence is one of the most potent open-ended questions in your repertoire.

Encourage clients to be specific about issues. This helps them know what you want to hear. If a patient has described an erectile failure experience, you can encourage detail and specificity by a question like, 'I know you felt tense when you got into bed with Sue and couldn't get an erection.

BOX 5-2

Non-verbal indicators of listening

1. Face the client squarely. (While this applies to general counselling, it can—as mentioned in previous chapters—be too confronting for sexual counselling, and sitting at a 90-degree angle is preferred.)
2. Adopt an open posture. Crossed legs and arms signal that you are defensive.
3. Lean towards the client.
4. Maintain good eye contact. This does not mean that you should stare at the client, but it does suggest that you look at the client when he or she is talking.
5. Try to relax.

Derived from: Egan, G. *The skilled helper. Models, skills and methods of effective helping.* (2nd edn). Monterey: Brooks/Cole, 1982.

Was there something about the situation that started you off feeling that way?'.

Reflecting back what the client has said is also helpful. First, it shows that you have been listening. Secondly, it acts as a check that you have understood accurately what has been said. A patient describes inhibitions resulting from parents-in-law being in the next bedroom. 'Right, so you feel uncomfortable that they might hear you, huh?'

Accurate empathy

Empathy is the ability to see the world from the client's perspective. This implies an understanding of what the client has experienced and how he or she reacted emotionally. Not only do you need to be able to see the world from the client's point of view, but you need to communicate your understanding.

Again, summarizing and reflecting back are excellent ways of communicating your willingness to see things from the client's point of view.

REFERENCES

1. Rogers, C.R. *Client-centered therapy.* Boston: Houghton Mifflin, 1951.
2. Rogers, C.R. *On becoming a person.* Boston: Houghton Mifflin, 1961.

3. Rogers, C.R. The necessary and sufficient conditions of therapeutic personality change. *Journal of Consulting Psychology*, 1957; 21: 95–104.

4. Packard, V. *The sexual wilderness*. London: Longmans, Green and Company, 1968.

5. Egan, G. *The skilled helper. Models, skills and methods of effective helping*. (6th edn). Monterey: Brooks/Cole, 1997.

6. Nelson-Jones, R. *Practical Counselling and Helping Skills*. (4th edn). London: Cassell, 1996.

7. Johnson, A.M., Wadsworth, J., Wellings, K., Field, J. and Bradshaw, S. *Sexual attitudes and lifestyles*. Oxford: Blackwell, 1994.

8. Janus, S.S and Janus, C.L. *The Janus report on sexual behavior*. New York: John Wiley, 1993.

6 *Sexual counselling and treatment*

This chapter outlines the PLISSIT model of sexual counselling.[1] It also suggests interventions for some of the more commonly encountered dysfunctions. A brief guide to sexual dysfunction is given in Stedman.[2]

THE PLISSIT MODEL

The PLISSIT model suggests that interventions in sexual dysfunctions can occur at four levels of complexity.

Box 6-1 outlines the levels of intervention.

Permission

At this level the practitioner introduces questions about the patient's sexuality (or, more rarely, responds to sexual questions or information volunteered by the patient). These actions establish that it is totally appropriate to discuss sexual matters in a professional setting, and that the practitioner is able and willing to clarify the issues involved and to initiate treatment if necessary. Annon[1] notes that many patients are able to develop their own plan to address their sexual concerns just by having a safe place in which to discuss sexual issues. Across the spectrum, probably the most common sexual concern is that of 'normality'. Is it normal to masturbate? Is it normal for my child to be doing X at this age? Are my genitals/breasts normal? Is it normal to occasionally fantasize, do . . ., etc.? Providing permission for patients to verbalize their concern and giving reassurance, where appropriate, that their issue is a common human concern, can provide much relief and even resolve their problem.

Limited information

Sometimes, brief information may be all that is needed. For example, depending on the patient's presenting concern, the following information can be helpful:

BOX 6-1
The PLISSIT model

- Permission to talk about sexual matters, fantasize, enjoy sexuality
- Limited Information
- Specific Suggestions
- Intensive Therapy

Derived from: Annon, J.S. *The behavioral treatment of sexual problems: brief therapy.* Honolulu: Enabling Systems, 1974.

- Many women take longer than men to warm up sexually. There is a need for protracted foreplay, starting with non-genital contact.
- Most women also take longer to cool down than men. Rolling over and going to sleep immediately after ejaculation is simply not good enough.
- Many women do not reach orgasm during penetrative intercourse (although this does not necessarily mean that they don't enjoy it).
- Many men find direct genital stimulation pleasurable and arousing even before they have attained an erection.
- Most men (over 18 years) require some physical stimulation to the penis to achieve a full erection.
- Occasional same-sex fantasies are common for persons of all sexual orientations.
- Many women find direct stimulation of the clitoris highly unpleasant if they have not reached a state of sexual arousal. Ouch.
- People differ in the level of their sex drives and this affects most noticeably the frequency of intercourse they would ideally like.[3]

Another important area of limited information concerns the possible effects of medication on erectile functioning. Physicians are sometimes reluctant to warn male patients that a drug may reduce erectile capacity. They believe that a man may expect failure, become anxious and thus induce erectile functioning difficulties. Similarly, with both men and women, some physicians may overlook informing patients of effects of drugs on libido. Neglecting such information can cause harm to individuals and their relationships. Where sexual side effects of drugs are common, it is better to inform patients about this, as well as indicating a plan of action should this occur (e.g., substituting another drug or lowering the dosage). This increases the probability that patients will report back if they are having problems rather than just accepting the situation or taking themselves off the medication.

The PLISSIT model emphasizes that providing limiting information means answering the specific question(s) and concerns of the patients, not of the physician. Thus, for patients having difficulty using condoms, it can be faster and more effective to ask them what specific difficulties they have, rather than launching into a general patient information session on condom use.

Specific suggestions

In the PLISSIT model, specific suggestions refer to brief therapy using behavioral exercises to address specific concerns. Some exercises, for example the sensate focus exercises or Kegel exercises, can be used in a wide variety of situations. Others, such as the squeeze technique in premature ejaculation, have a more specialized application. These suggestions are discussed later in this chapter.

Intensive therapy

Some sexual concerns can only be effectively addressed by referral to a specialist sex therapist. Referral is indicated when there is major accompanying psychopathology, substance abuse, risk to others (e.g., sex offending), sexual identity concerns, major relationship discord, or in any case when the primary practitioner feels out of his or her depth.

Referral

There are two opposing considerations to be weighed in the balance when you are considering referring a patient to a specialist sex therapist. Certainly, the patient may receive more sophisticated and perhaps longer term treatment. On the other hand, it is easy for the patient to perceive referral as rejection and/or further pathologization. 'I must really be sick if my doctor wants me to see a specialist.' Especially for the patient who has had difficulties and doubts about mentioning sexual matters, it may seem as if he or she has overstepped the mark of acceptability. Hence, sensitivity should be exercised when making referrals for sexual concerns. Providing patients with options can be a respectful way of assisting the patient to seek help: 'Some of my patients with this concern like to start by doing some reading on this topic, others prefer to have a referral to a therapist with specialized training . . . What would work best for you?'.

SEXUAL DISORDERS

In the Diagnostic and Statistical Manual (DSM-IV) sexual disorders are subdivided into three categories: dysfunctions (grouped according to the sexual response cycle), paraphilias and gender identity disorders. This chapter deals with the diagnosis and treatment of the first group: the sexual dysfunctions.

Treating sexual dysfunctions

Treating sexual dysfunctions can be one of the most interesting parts of sexual counselling. Careful diagnosis, appropriate intervention and regular monitoring sessions are essential features of good treatment. For any sexual dysfunction, at least four possible causes exist that may explain the dysfunction: patient characteristics (both organic and psychogenic causes), partner characteristics (including concurrent dysfunction), relationship characteristics (commonly inability to communicate sexually) and situational or other characteristics that prevent successful functioning. The practitioner should examine each of these as part of initial assessment and diagnosis.

Behavioral interventions

Where there is not an obvious organic cause of the sexual dysfunction, behavioral intervention, such as treating with sensate focus exercises, is the first line of treatment. Even when organic causes are suspected, these exercises can still be helpful in increasing sexual activity. These can be employed in a wide variety of situations, if necessary modifying the rules to fit the specific situation. Sensate focus exercises allow the couple to re-learn how to have sex by focussing on their own bodies and their responses. They can be used to enhance sexual enjoyment in a situation where no dysfunction exists, in orgasmic dysfunction, in premature and retarded ejaculation, and so on. Box 6-2 gives a summary of the exercises, but fuller accounts are given by Masters and Johnson[4] and Kaplan.[5]

The exercises have many uses:

- To enable people to get to know their own and their partner's preferred placing, timing and kind of tactile stimulation
- To enable sexually anxious people to relax with each other
- To reduce pressure to perform
- As part of a planned dysfunction treatment program.

BOX 6-2
Sensate focus exercises

The couple lie together naked on a comfortable surface where they can ensure privacy (even if it means fitting a bolt to the door). One partner lies on his or her stomach while the other systematically strokes him or her from the back of the head to the toes, taking time over each body part. The role of the stroker is to experiment with different kinds of touching, that of the receiver to focus on enjoyment of body responses and to give a little feedback about what he or she finds pleasurable.

When either partner chooses, the receiver turns over and the partner begins sensual fondling of the front of the body, avoiding the breasts and genitals. (Most authorities confine themselves to suggesting avoiding a female's breasts, but male nipples can be highly charged erogenous zones too.)

When either partner decides, the roles are reversed. The rules at this stage are simple:

- No genital or nipple touching
- No intercourse
- Tell your partner what you like (and what you don't)
- Don't rush.

The partners are asked to carry out the exercise two or three times before their next appointment with the practitioner. When both partners are ready, they may include nipple and genital touching, but the rule about no intercourse continues.

It may happen in either of the two first stages that one or both partners becomes sexually aroused. If so, they should masturbate afterwards, alone if that can be arranged. Again, when both partners are good and ready, they can progress to intercourse, but without any pressure to reach orgasm.

Derived from: Masters, W.H. and Johnson, V.E. *Human sexual inadequacy.* Boston: Little, Brown and Company, 1970.

The exercises are typically given as 'homework'. Couples are asked to try them out two or three times between sessions. They then discuss their responses to the exercises in the therapy period.

The couple move gradually through the exercises at their own pace. In the beginning, stimulation of genitals and breasts is off-limits. When the two people are comfortable with this level, they move along to genital touching, but with intercourse still prohibited.

The practitioner and couple together decide the level at which they can comfortably start. Very sexually anxious people are encouraged to begin by lying down fully clothed and then kissing and cuddling.

One of the most controversial aspects of sensate focus exercises for many couples is the 'intercourse ban'. While the couple are learning new ways of pleasuring through their exercises, they are asked to abstain from the old behavioral patterns, in particular attempting intercourse. The intercourse ban can be a very informative exercise for couples as it forces them to discuss how much they want intercourse, what it means to them, and what life would be like without intercourse. For many couples it is also a paradoxical intervention. By outlawing intercourse, many patients come back reporting their first experiences of intercourse in months.

Except for treating premature ejaculation, where oil increases sensation, we see no reason not to use massage oil in these exercises. There are many varieties of oil on the market, or cold-pressed almond oil with a dash of scented herb oil is also good.

An important component of the exercises is to discourage what Masters and Johnson[4] call 'spectatoring'; that is, the anxious monitoring of one's sexual functioning, worries about how the partner is responding, and so on. Addressing anxiety, and specifically asking the couple how they can take the performance pressure off themselves, is important.

A note on terminology here. When treating sexual dysfunctions, it is more accurate, helpful and respectful to define the problem as behavioral. Avoid terms like 'premature ejaculator', 'impotent' or 'frigid' which frame sexual functioning as an identity concern. Hence, a patient is not a 'retarded ejaculator who is impotent' but rather a person 'having a problem with maintaining erections to the point of achieving ejaculation'. Similarly, the term 'psychogenic' is unfortunate: many patients will think you are implying they're 'wrong', 'sick' or 'psycho'. Pointing out that 'sexual dysfunction' means simply a problem in sexual behavior functioning avoids blame, and helps prepare the patient to discuss a behavioral modification plan.

In the next section we look at specific sexual dysfunctions and approaches to treatment.

Sexual desire discrepancy

Perhaps the most common sexual concern of patients is sexual desire discrepancy, where one or other partner will present complaining about the lack of sex in the relationship, while the other complains about the sexual demands of the partner and how it is turning her or him off. Frequently, a patient will present seeking help for his or her partner, who is identified as 'frigid' or 'impotent'. On coming in, the partner reports that everything is fine except for her or his 'hypersexual' partner! Often one partner may think she or he is turning the other partner on, while the other partner is in fact being turned off. Another common pattern is for one partner to be wanting more loving 'non-sexual' touch and affirmation, while the other is feeling sexually frustrated and rejected. Both become withholding in the hope that the other recognizes what each wants. Sexual desire discrepancy can be very destructive to the relationship and to the self-esteem of both partners. If left untreated, it can result in either the break-up of the relationship or years of frustration and bitterness.

The first step in treating sexual desire discrepancy is to interview both partners. It is important to interview partners separately regarding their own perception of whether they have a sexual problem, their sexual desires, history of abuse and/or negative experiences, current behavior (including secrets they may not have shared with their partner) and goals for treatment. Where hypoactive sexual desire or compulsive sexual behavior patterns are substantiated, treatment for these concerns should be recommended. Then, interview the partners together to establish common goals for treatment and what an acceptable sexual and emotional life relationship would look like for each partner. Where one partner has an identified sexual dysfunction, this can then be treated. Otherwise couples counselling is indicated. Pointing out that differences in desire are entirely normal, and helping each partner to negotiate an acceptable plan to enhance the relationship, will be helpful. Comments reinforcing sexual stereotypes—'men always want sex anyway', and 'women don't like sex'—only reinforce the problem, and are best avoided. Setting mutual goals does not mean that both partners always have to settle for compromise. Dr Bean Robinson[6] has published a helpful exercise, 'My week, your week', as an alternative to compromise (see Box 6-3).

Hypoactive sexual desire disorder and sexual aversion disorder

Some people report a persistent absence of or aversion to sex, even in the area of fantasies and desire for sexual activity. The first step in such cases is

BOX 6-3

My week, your week

This exercise required the couple to agree on three things.

The first step is for the couple to negotiate boundaries: what activities are mutually acceptable and how often. This may require the partner who is more 'shut down' to identify behaviors that they could engage in under the right circumstances.

Second, both then agree that for the sake of the relationship they will mutually abide by the rules with grace and good humor, and make good faith attempts to support their partner.

Third, the couple establish a schedule where on partner 1's week, partner 1 is responsible for prioritizing and initiating sex and emotional interactions at whatever frequency partner 1 prefers (within the limits negotiated in step 1). Partner 1's job is to nurture the relationship's sex life. Partner 2's job is to be responsive. The roles are then reversed during partner 2's week.

to take a full medical and sexual history to identify possible contributors. Physical (e.g., hypothyroidism) and pharmacologic causes should be ruled out prior to assuming the problem is psychosexual. Referral to a specialist can be helpful; otherwise graduated exercises for hypoactive sexual desire and systematic desensitization exercises for sexual aversion are indicated.

Compulsive sexual behavior

At the other end of the continuum to hypoactive sexual desire disorder is preoccupation with and compulsive seeking of sex. Historically defined as hypersexuality, hyperphilia, Don Juanism and sexual addiction, compulsive sexual behavior remains controversial, principally because of confusion with healthy sexual drive. Compulsive sexual behavior is distinct from a healthy interest in sex and from adolescent sexual maturation (see chapter 14) and experimentation during the coming out process (see chapter 13), all of which may include lots of sexual activity but not be compulsive. Compulsive sexual behavior should be considered when sexual preoccupation and/or activity clearly has negative medical, legal, financial, psychological, social or other significant daily impact on the patient's functioning (e.g., a pattern of STDs, loss of employment and relationships from sexual

BOX 6-4

Questions to ask to identify patients with compulsive sexual behavior

1. Do you or others who know you find that you are overly preoccupied or obsessed with sexual activity?
2. Do you ever find youself compelled to engage in sexual activity in response to stress, anxiety or depression?
3. Have you had serious problems develop as a result of your sexual behavior?
4. Do you feel guilty and shameful about some of your sexual behaviors?
5. Do you fantasize or engage in any unusual or what some would consider 'deviant' sexual behavior?
6. Do you ever find yourself sexually obsessed with someone who is not interested in you or doesn't even know you?
7. Have you had numerous love relationships that are short-lived, intense and unfulfilling?
8. Do you feel a constant need for sex or expressions of love in your sexual relationship?

Derived from: Coleman, E. Is your patient suffering from compulsive sexual behavior? *Psychiatric Annals*, 1992; 22(6): 320–325.

preoccupation, arrest for sex-related behavior, and intense guilt and shame).

Compulsive sexual behavior is defined as behavior driven by anxiety-reduction mechanisms rather than sexual desire. The behavior may be normophilic (e.g., masturbation) or paraphilic (e.g., exhibitionism). Obsessive thoughts and compulsive rituals reduce anxiety and distress, but they create a self-perpetuating cycle. In addition, there is high comorbidity with anxiety disorders, depression, and alcohol and drug dependence. In the past decade clinical research has made significant progress in developing successful treatment (usually involving some combination of group therapy and pharmacotherapy). Practitioners interested in learning more about diagnosing and treating compulsive sexual behavior should consult Coleman's article, 'Is your patient suffering from compulsive sexual behavior?'.[7] Box 6-4 details questions to identify patients with compulsive sexual behavior.

Erectile dysfunction

Having decided that the causes of erectile dysfunction are not organic (see chapter 3), you need to determine what psychological factors are, or have been, operating. We say, 'or have been' because sometimes a single episode of erectile failure produces anxiety at the next attempt. This reduces the chance of a functional erection and a vicious cycle is set up. By reviewing the original episode with the patient, salient factors that induced the erection difficulties can be recognized and treated.

All kinds of things can trigger off a failure experience. One patient described the super-tidy flat of his mistress-to-be. 'Even her jumpers were all folded up in those little basket things. I just couldn't get it up.'

Common factors include the patient's own concerns, partner characteristics, the relationship and the situation (see Box 6-5). When a psychological cause (or causes) is found, it should be directly treated. The permission level of the PLISSIT model is important as the practitioner encourages the patient to tease out the components that led to erectile failure in the first place. It is also helpful to provide limited information about the feedback loop, where anxiety leads to a greater chance of failure, and about the role of spectatoring.

The role of the counsellor is to help the patient identify the factors that triggered off the original failure experience. If those components are still present, what can be done? A sexually passive partner may be encouraged to take a more active role, while a sexually active partner may be encouraged to let her or his partner take the lead. Bolts can be fitted to bedroom doors. The occasional visit to a motel can be undertaken. All sorts of minor, practical adjustments can be made.

Perhaps the most salient intervention is to initiate sensate focus exercises with a co-operative and attractive partner. When the man finds that he can enjoy sensual experiences with no pressure to proceed to intercourse, there is a good chance that he will begin to have erections again. If his partner is female, the woman-on-top position is possibly the easiest way to re-start intercourse. It does not necessarily require a full erection and is easier to incorporate into sensate focus exercises. Even when a physician may suspect the sexual dysfunction is not primarily a behavioral concern, it may be necessary for couples to first try the exercises before they are ready to address more complex reasons for sexual incompatibility.

Chemical interventions

Viagra is the first of several new drugs that radically improve erectile capacity in a high proportion of men. In most countries, it must be prescribed

BOX 6-5
Triggers for erectile difficulties

Features of the man
- Anxiety about previous failures
- Spectatoring tendency

Features of the partner
- A partner of the non-preferred sex
- A partner who is not attractive to the man (obesity, aging, not good looking, inverted nipples, etc.)
- A moody, cross, irritable, tense or preoccupied partner
- A passive, unenthusiastic or unwilling partner

Features of the relationship
- Poor communication skills
- Differences in sexual desire, drive and other differences between the partners
- Differences in preferred activities and sexual priorities

Features of the situation
- Lack of privacy, possibility of interruption
- Guilt about infidelity
- Desire to impress a new partner
- Overuse of drugs or alcohol
- Medication effects
- Alertness for crying children

by a medical practitioner. Before prescribing Viagra it is important to complete a detailed erectile difficulties history, as Viagra is not an appropriate intervention where partner, relationship and/or situational factors are the identified problem. In providing patient education on Viagra, physicians should be clear that even with Viagra, a man will still need to have physical stimulation to get and maintain an erection.

The most serious complication of using Viagra is a synergistic effect, especially for patients on antihypertensive medication and people who use nitrites (poppers) during sex, resulting in a dramatic and potentially lethal drop in blood pressure. Hence, prior to prescribing Viagra, a physician must ask about what other medications the patient is using, and whether the person ever uses nitrites (poppers). Other minor but still serious side effects include dilation of blood vessels which can result in headache or prolonged penile erection (priapism). Because many men with erectile difficulties imagine that a prolonged erection would be heavenly, it is wise to educate patients that erections lasting three to four hours can be painful and cause damage, and advise them to seek emergency room help should priapism occur.

It should be noted that other oral pharmacotherapies are currently in the research and development phase.

Any change, even improvements in patterns of sexual intercourse, can impact on the relationship both positively and negatively. In most cases, both partners may be delighted at the resumption or enhancement of their sexual activity. Men taking Viagra commonly report decreased anxiety about maintaining erections, while both partners note they can relax more, confident that the man will be able to get and maintain an erection sufficient for intercourse. But for a significant number of couples, the reintroduction of sexual intercourse (through Viagra or other interventions) can have unanticipated side effects. Some partners resent any change to the status quo, others have adjusted happily to reduced or absent sexual activity in the relationship, while still others may feel, 'It's not him making love to me; it's just the drug'. Physicians can help to minimize these negative effects by mentioning such potential outcomes prior to prescribing oral pharmacotherapy. Both partners should be consulted if they have any reservations about its use. A follow-up consultation, again with both partners, can be therapeutic.

Surgical prophylaxes

In cases of organically based dysfunction or psychogenic dysfunction that does not respond to treatment (relatively rare), surgical implants may be considered. This usually necessitates referral to a urological surgeon.

Premature ejaculation

Defining premature ejaculation can be difficult. Usually, the best operational definition is the fact that the patient and/or his partner are concerned enough to bring it to a physician's attention. Typically, premature ejaculation occurs because the man is anxious and/or doesn't recognize when he is about to ejaculate. This can occur either because the man is inexperienced in recognizing his own body's reactions or because he becomes so focussed on his partner that he loses his awareness of himself. Regardless of cause, premature ejaculation is relatively easy to treat and the prognosis is

---

BOX 6-6
A failure of communication

Mr D.'s preferred technique for delaying orgasm was to recite the teams of the English Football League to himself, beginning with the lowest division. He would utter early warning signals from time to time. ('I'm up to Charlton Athletic, love.') He would eventually collapse, with a triumphant cry of, 'Liverpool!'.

He and his wife, who was not orgasmic with intercourse, had seemingly never discussed this behavior. Mr D. was upset about the dysfunction and rather angry considering his heroic efforts.

In a conjoint session, Mrs D. volunteered that she would prefer him to come at any time he chose, as she didn't find intercourse stimulating anyway. During intercourse she tended to plan meals and shopping for the following week.

Therapy focussed on sexual enjoyment and increased foreplay, with Mrs D. reaching orgasm before intercourse started.

---

almost always excellent. Behavioral questioning of how long a patient typically lasts (specific to vaginal, oral and anal intercourse and in masturbation), whether intromission can occur, and the patient's expectation of how he should be able to perform can verify the diagnosis, as well as the specificity and severity of the condition. Because expectations can be unrealistic, it is essential to ask about the length of time. A patient who was asked to be more specific about his problem answered, 'After quarter of an hour or so, I just can't stop it'.

Many men take their own initiatives to delay ejaculation. Box 6-6 gives a rather disastrous example of this approach. It also illustrates the need for communication between sexual partners.

There are two major categories of behavioral treatment. One, aimed at increased ejaculatory control, can be described as the 'P.E.'s a disease' approach. The other is designed to allow the couple to enjoy their sexual experiences without focussing on ejaculation.

While many couples want to prolong intercourse, the second approach is quicker, easier and relatively fail-safe.

The usual approaches to enhancing ejaculatory control involve some combination of three techniques:

- Graded sensate focus exercises
- Semans'[9] technique
- Masters and Johnson's[4] squeeze technique.

The initial step, as always, is permission. The partners need permission to talk about their experiences. They also need permission to enjoy sensuality and sexuality, especially where one or both have guilt feelings about sex. Normalizing is also helpful. Informing the patient that most men, especially when young, experience premature ejaculation from time to time, can help relieve patients' anxieties.

Providing some limited information about premature ejaculation can be helpful. Some men have never used their hand to masturbate. In such cases, providing permission for the man to pleasure himself in order to recognize when he is approaching the point of inevitability can be helpful. Practising modified Kegel exercises can assist the patient both to learn more about ejaculatory control and to recognize his own body's responses. Informing couples that most men ejaculate within two minutes of intromission can assist in relieving pressure to last forever.[6] The patient can be reassured, however, that if he and his partner are willing to co-operate, he can learn to delay ejaculation. At this point, taking a full sexual history of both patients can be helpful. Many men with premature ejaculation concerns present as both less experienced in knowing their own body and its sexual signals, as well as less confident in having sex with a partner. Other men may have a history of early experience of situations where it was important to come quickly (furtive masturbation, danger of invasion of privacy, use of workers in the sex industry for whom time is money, etc.) or where sex was particularly anxious. Taking this history can help both physician and patient to understand how the behavioral pattern developed and became maintained.

Specific suggestions

Initially, a graded set of sensate focus exercises combined with Semans' technique can be outlined (see Box 6-7). The couple should try to do the exercises at least twice in the week before the next appointment.

We need to say a word about sexual satisfaction of both partners in the early stages of the program. It is better, if it is acceptable to them, that they masturbate in private after finishing the exercises if they feel the need.

Certainly, the program is very demanding, especially for the partner. You need to be completely honest about this before people begin, as failure experiences can be both demoralizing and destructive.

You also need to tell the couple that in the early stages of the program,

BOX 6-7
Semans' technique and sensate focus exercises

The couple lie naked together and the patient's partner touches the patient's body, avoiding the genitals and nipples, until he gets an erection. The partner continues stimulation until the man signals that he is close to ejaculation. The partner then ceases stimulation until the ejaculatory urge (and perhaps the erection) subsides. The partner then begins again and repeats the procedure two or three times.

The instructions given to the man are that he should be totally and utterly selfish. He focusses on his own sensual and sexual responses and on telling his partner when he begins to feel the ejaculatory urge.

Once the couple can manage this step satisfactorily, they move on to a similar procedure that now involves genital and nipple stimulation. Again, the partner ceases stimulation when the man signals the ejaculatory urge.

In later sessions, when the patient gains a firm erection, he inserts it into his partner, but does not make any pelvic movements. At the ejaculatory urge, he withdraws and lies quietly until the urge subsides. This is repeated two or three times.

The next step is to incorporate slight pelvic thrusting, but again to withdraw at the start of the ejaculatory urge.

Rationale

This program is rather similar to Wolpe and Lazarus's[10] systematic desensitization technique for the treatment of phobias. There, progressively stronger phobic stimuli are introduced when the patient is in a state incompatible with anxiety, such as relaxation. The program allows the man to become more aware of his sexual responses, especially those relating to ejaculation, and gradually deconditions the early ejaculation behavior.

when the man is less in tune with the sensations leading up to ejaculation, he may accidentally come. If this happens, they should simply suspend operations for a while.

The Masters and Johnson[4] squeeze technique can be used as a quick means of suppressing the ejaculatory urge. (For some reason most books illustrate this by a hand with dangerously long fingernails.) When the patient feels the ejaculatory urge, his partner grasps his penis firmly, thumb on the frenum, first two fingers on the head of the penis, and squeezes. It's a good idea for the patient to give feedback about the amount of pressure to be used. Most partners are initially reluctant to squeeze hard enough. Warn the couple that the patient's erection will probably subside to a degree.

Other approaches

Many couples with sexual functioning concerns find the strict behavioral modification regimen employed by sensate focus unacceptable, and either disobey the rules, modify them, or adapt them to their own situation. It's important to see each couple's situation as unique, and deal with their particular concerns.

Not all couples need to have intercourse to be sexually satisfied. Contrary to popular belief, many women—and especially those who tend not to be orgasmic through vaginal intercourse—do not particularly enjoy vaginal intercourse (see Box 6-6). Helping such couples to give themselves permission to validate their preferred methods of lovemaking is helpful. For these couples, therapy can focus on enhancing enjoyment of sexual relations without the rigorous re-learning of ejaculatory control.

There are several specific suggestions that can enhance a couple's sexual enjoyment. Give them a choice.

- *Bibliotherapy:* Buy a good guide to sex. For heterosexual couples, nothing in our opinion has outshone Comfort's *The joy of sex.*[11] Silverstein and White's *The joy of gay sex*[12] is a good manual for gay men. Loulan's sensitive books on women's sex with women are a good guide.[13,14]
- *Patient education:* Spend a session with them explaining the physiology of sexual arousal, plateau, recognizing point of inevitability, mechanisms of orgasm, and so forth. Like those with anxiety disorders, many men with premature ejaculation cope by avoiding their concerns. Simple education can both reassure the patient and address gaps in education.
- *Partner focus:* Make sure the partner comes, by manual, oral or any other congenial form of stimulation, before the patient inserts his penis. Have the patient stimulate his partner almost to orgasm, insert his penis, lie still and continue to stimulate the partner.

- *Physical intervention:* Use condoms, especially ones with ribs and 'ticklers'. The reduced sensation can often delay male orgasm. Similarly, some creams are marketed to assist men to last longer. Typically these work by having a mild numbing effect on the penis.
- *Modified behavioral intervention:* After explaining sensate focus, it can be helpful to have the couple develop their own modified form of sensate focus. Play sensate focus games with relaxed rules.
- *Vacation days:* For couples where sex has always been difficult, discuss whether they wish to insert 'vacation days' into their overall plan, where they can just be sexual.
- *Reframing the symptom:* Some people may suggest that the patient ejaculates quickly, once, 'to get the premature ejaculation over and done with' and then continues lovemaking using the refractory period. However, we have had many men with this precise pattern present still very frustrated at the premature ejaculation.

Pharmacotherapy

Many men with sexual function concerns desire a 'magic pill' to make their particular condition disappear. As with Viagra for erectile difficulties, several antidepressants commonly have the side effect of delaying ejaculation, and hence can be used to treat premature ejaculation. They are good tools for brief interventions and will either alleviate the problem or illuminate it. However, the physician needs to examine the costs and benefits of providing such medications. In situations where the premature ejaculation is clearly secondary to a generalized depressive or anxiety disorder, medication can be helpful in treating the overall condition. However, medication is not always the best intervention. In the absence of such disorders, medication sends the powerful message to the already anxious man that his problem is medical (not behavioral). Medication typically also lowers libido and over time can lead to retarded ejaculation. When considering medication, practitioners should consider the long-term as well as short-term outcomes. Unnecessary use of medication to treat a problem that can be treated as successfully or more successfully using less invasive techniques should be discouraged.

Retarded ejaculation

Much retarded ejaculation results from medication side effects. As we said, it is really only fair to warn the patient of this possibility when the drug is prescribed. This warning is the equivalent of *permission* to discuss any sexual problems that may arise from using the drug. If problems do arise, the need is to balance therapeutic gains against side effects, with due reference to the

73

needs of the patient. A related drug may not affect ejaculation. A lower dosage may be sufficient for clinical gains.

Medications (notably some antipsychotics) may also produce dry ejaculation. Semen enters the bladder rather than the urethra. The same balancing of priorities and considerations of alternatives apply.

Through accidents, medically necessary surgery, and disability, the patient may face permanent impotence, inability to ejaculate, inability to orgasm, or some combination of these. This does not mean the person ceases to be a sexual being, however. Studies of rehabilitation have shown that while most physicians tend to focus on assisting the patient to return to work, most patients' primary concern is whether they can be sexual again. Even in situations of paraplegia where the patient may have little or no physical sensations, the psychological importance of sexual pleasuring is well recognized. Counselling of a supportive nature, discussing the importance of pleasuring to each partner, and *specific suggestions* where the physician and patient discuss modified sexual activities that fit the patient's circumstances, are important.

As with all sexual concerns, the first step is to take an adequate history to confirm the retarded ejaculation and to investigate cause. As with premature ejaculation in younger men, some occasional retarded ejaculation in older men is entirely normal, in which case normalizing this for the patient and providing reassurance is all that is required. Where a significant pattern of retarded ejaculation is confirmed (atypical for the patient's age and health), in addition to medical concerns, we would recommend referral to a specialist sex therapist. The complex interaction of sexual, emotional and situational factors takes more time and expertise to analyse and work through than is available in most general health care situations.

If referral is not an option, say in a remote country practice, we suggest that you start by finding out when the man can ejaculate, if at all; when was his last ejaculation; and whether he can identify any reasons for not being able to ejaculate. It is helpful to ascertain whether the retarded ejaculation is situation-specific or pervasive. While some men may be able to confirm if they can ejaculate, usually through masturbation, many others for various reasons neither masturbate nor attempt sex with their partner(s). In such situations, providing permission to masturbate and setting 'self-pleasuring' for homework may be necessary in order to clarify organicity or psychogenic cause. Where the retarded ejaculation is specific to intercourse, many men and their partners fear this means they no longer find their partner attractive. Hence both partners may be feeling guilty, 'un-sexy' and fear their relationship is under threat. From the physiological stand-point, the most common cause of retarded ejaculation is lack of sufficient friction to the penis to reach the point of inevitability. Explaining this to the patient or couple, and asking directly about the degree of stimulation to the penis in intercourse, will be necessary.

Frequently, erectile difficulties and retarded ejaculation occur together. Where erectile capacity is present sufficient for intercourse, sensate focus exercises can be helpful. Start with the patient masturbating himself alone to reassure himself that he can ejaculate. Then, in the presence of his partner, he can masturbate, explaining as he proceeds what sort of touch/friction his penis enjoys. Eventually the partner's hand is placed over the patient's hand as he masturbates. The couple progress to masturbation with the partner's hand alone. Once masturbation by the partner is achieved, the couple can proceed through the sensate focus exercises to intercourse if they wish.

The way men masturbate typically varies for each man, and varies across time and situations, and at different stages in the sexual response cycle. A man may start out needing long, slow strokes from the shaft to the head, modified to the shaft only as the head becomes more sensitive, culminating in fast stimulation of the whole penis as ejaculation nears. Explaining this to the couple highlights the need for the patient to show his partner how he typically likes to masturbate, what sort of touch he prefers, and how that varies. Because each man is different, even in gay male couples where one or both partners are experiencing sexual concerns, it is necessary for partners to become comfortable showing and telling each other what sort of pleasure they enjoy, and in particular, what sort of touching and stroking feels most pleasurable. Approached in a sensitive way, this exercise can lead to renewed intimacy and communication for both partners.

Female orgasmic dysfunction (anorgasmia and generalized orgasmic dysfunction)

The first need is to check whether the woman is only non-orgasmic during intercourse or whether she has orgasms during other activities such as masturbation, manual or oral stimulation or erotic dreams. As with men, the first step is to establish clear and realistic goals, and to provide *permission* for the woman to pleasure herself in order to learn about her body.

In early stages of treating anorgasmia, masturbation can be a difficulty for many women. Many women received very strong and powerful messages growing up that 'good' women do not masturbate; they feel sexually 'shut down', and hence are reluctant to masturbate. The practitioner needs to be sensitive to these barriers, and must work with the patient to set gradual goals. Even the term 'masturbation' can sound dirty or disgusting to some patients. Framing masturbation as 'self-pleasuring' can be helpful. As a health practitioner, pointing out that masturbation is perfectly normal, and even necessary to address the patient's concerns, can be part of providing permission. The Kinsey Report on female sexuality[15] found that over half of the sample masturbated. Masturbation may also be a positive health benefit. The increased flow of blood to the genitals in masturbation and intercourse helps maintain the vaginal epithelium, especially in postmenopausal women. It may also enhance orgasmic capacity.

For women who have never masturbated to orgasm, the program should start gently. A non-threatening beginning to learning about body responses is to focus on them in the shower. Encourage the woman to use a good shower gel or exfoliating cream. She gets wet, turns off the shower and then smoothes the cream over her body, paying attention to the sensuality of the experience and her bodily sensations.

One of the authors (LDC-L) finds that a productive, permission-giving approach is to use imagery in hypnosis. The woman is encouraged to imagine the scene as vividly as possible, 'almost as if you were really there'. Non-sexual images should be evoked, for example the luxury of sitting up in bed on a sunny morning and stretching every muscle, or feeling the warm sun and the texture of the sand as she lies on a beach, or the shower scene. The woman is encouraged to enjoy and be pleased with the feelings her body can produce. She can then move on at her own pace to genital touching without the aim of orgasm.

You can also point out that the myth of a distinction between vaginal and clitoral orgasms is just that—a myth.

Patients may find using sexual aids such as books and magazines helpful. Comfort's *The joy of sex*[11] is a sensible, warmly written guide. Loulan's books, *Lesbian sex*[13] and *Lesbian passion*[14] are useful for homosexual and bisexual women. (Not that heterosexuals cannot learn a lot from them too.) Working on fantasies is also helpful. Fantasies such as semi-public lovemaking (e.g., surreptitious stimulation under the tablecloth at a dinner party) and making love outdoors, are common female fantasies which can increase arousal. Nancy Friday's books on women's fantasies, *My Secret Garden*[16] and *Forbidden Flowers*,[17] are excellent homework reading both for educating women about other women's sexual fantasies and to assist patients to recognize their own fantasies.

A vibrator or other devices that enable a women to pleasure herself without manual stimulation can be a good place to start, although the woman will need to progress to manual stimulation eventually. The woman should masturbate two or three times a week in a situation where she is comfortable. She needs to focus on what kinds of body stimulation are pleasurable to her.

Providing *limited information* on sexual physiology is also important. Explaining that the majority of women do not reach orgasm during intercourse unless there is some direct stimulation of the clitoris, normalizes the patient's experience. You can tell the couple that female orgasm is caused by stimulation of the clitoris, an organ very like a small penis. It is important that the woman be aroused sexually by non-genital touching, kissing and cuddling before her partner touches her clitoris. It is downright unpleasant to be touched directly on an unaroused clitoris. It has been estimated that the 'average' woman takes about 45 minutes from the initiation of foreplay to orgasm. Could the couple be rushing things?

As part of homework, suggest to the patient that she take a mirror and examine her genitals. To know her own anatomy can be important for a woman who may be unaware or avoidant of sex.

Then, *specific suggestions* for graduated homework exercises can be set which enable the woman to experience her sexual functioning to orgasm. These usually start with the woman learning about her body alone, then teaching what she has learned about her body to her partner by guiding her partner's hand in masturbating her, then gradually reintroducing elements of sexual intercourse. As for men, one possibility is for the couple to accept that she is not going to reach orgasm easily in the intercourse situation. The couple can focus on plenty of foreplay, moving up to manual and oral stimulation of the clitoris, so that the woman reaches orgasm before intercourse begins. Because desire for intercourse frequently leads to perceived pressure on the woman to perform, the intercourse ban in early stages is very important. Setting the partner concurrent exercises to learn about her or his body also through masturbation can help provide the partner with permission to masturbate, decrease pressure to perform, and assist the patient not to feel that she is the total problem. While clitoral stimulation is the direct cause of orgasm, there are many possible inhibitors. Some of them are listed in Box 6-8.

Especially when women have breast-fed children, concurrent stimulation of a nipple and the clitoris may be exquisitely pleasurable. She should avoid spectatoring and the feeling that she *must* reach orgasm every time she masturbates. A water-soluble lubricant such as KY jelly may be useful in avoiding soreness.

When she is comfortable with masturbation, aware of what kinds of touching suit her and able to reach orgasm on at least some of the occasions, genital fondling may be incorporated into the sensate focus exercises

---

BOX 6-8

Factors inhibiting female orgasm

Features of the patient
- Guilt about sex
- Lack of knowledge and/or experience
- Anxiety and tension
- Anger and hostility
- Depression
- Tiredness
- Spectatoring
- Concerns about possible pregnancy
- Pelvic pain

Features of the situation
- Possibility of interruption
- Guilt about infidelity
- Alertness for crying children
- Physical discomfort (e.g., a small parked car)
- Distractions (e.g., noisy neighbours)
- Reluctance to have intercourse

Features of the partner
- Physically unattractive to the patient
- Poor sexual technique
- Sexual dysfunction
- Preferences for distasteful or uncomfortable acts
- Not the preferred sex

Features of the relationship
- Poor communication
- Partner pressure to perform
- Marital discord

---

if she chooses and her partner agrees. She should tell her partner about what pleases her, where she wants to be touched and how, then guide him or her in touching her. She can demonstrate what kind of touching works best. (Many partners are sexually aroused by the sight of a woman masturbating.)

For heterosexual couples, the next step is to initiate orgasm with the man's penis in the woman's vagina. As the woman nears orgasm she or he should stimulate the partner's penis to erection. She then straddles him as he continues to stimulate her and inserts his penis just as she reaches orgasm. The length of time of penis insertion can be gradually increased, still using the woman-on-top position, as this makes it easier for the man to continue direct clitoral stimulation when the penis is inserted.

For lesbian couples, there are few hard data on orgasmic dysfunction. We suspect that lesbian women may be relatively reluctant to present with sexual problems to a predominantly heterosexual and still rather male-dominated profession. In considering referrals for sexual concerns, a practitioner should inquire whether the therapist is both sensitive to lesbian couples' concerns and knowledgeable about female sexual dysfunction.

It is our impression that lesbian couples may have less orgasmic dysfunction than heterosexual couples. Our reasons for this opinion are as follows:

- So much of the limited information that proves to be therapeutic in counselling heterosexual couples is straightforward education about differences between men and women in terms of sexual response cycles. A woman can apply her knowledge of her own responses to the likely feelings of her female partner.
- Perhaps a woman would be more understanding of the fact that a female partner can enjoy sex without reaching orgasm. A fair proportion of women who are not orgasmic present on the insistence of their male partners who feel that they, the men, are failures if the woman does not reach orgasm.
- Oral and manual stimulation, major components in lesbian sexuality, are far more likely to lead to orgasm than is a short period of foreplay followed by intercourse.
- Other research suggests that lesbian couples, as a group, may be better than either heterosexual or gay male couples in prioritizing their relationships, discussing concerns and resolving difficulties.[18]

On the other hand, Loulan,[13] a lesbian sex therapist, describes orgasmic difficulties in her patients. They include:

- Anorgasmia
- Orgasm by masturbation, but not with a partner
- Differing response speed of the partners.

Loulan suggests masturbation practice and a variety of sensate focus style exercises. She also recommends that women remove themselves from what she calls the tyranny of orgasm as a goal in lovemaking. 'Orgasm is highly overrated.' This attitude of mind seems an excellent way to remove performance pressure and might well be incorporated into heterosexual therapy.

We suggest that you read Loulan's books[13,14] before treating a lesbian patient. You can also refer her to the homework exercises towards the end of the earlier book.

Vaginismus

Vaginismus is best treated by referral to a specialist sex therapist. Of course, this is not always possible.

The approach to vaginismus involves three aspects:

* Relaxation techniques
* Permission to enjoy sexuality and encouragement of this
* The insertion of progressively larger objects into the vagina.

We find that teaching the woman to relax, with or without hypnosis, is a useful beginning. The imagery suggested above for non-orgasmic women is appropriate.

Goldberg[19] suggests a structured program. The practitioner explains the rationale of the treatment using the analogy of lift phobia. It is essential to stress that the patient will be moving along at her own pace and will not be rushed.

Therapy will aim at change in three areas:

* Removal of the physical spasm of the muscles
* The woman's feelings of anxiety or resentment about penetration
* The woman's concerns that she is abnormal.

As homework, the woman listens to a hypnosis or relaxation tape in the morning. The tape contains sensual imagery of the kind we have described plus desensitizing imagery.

In the evening, she listens to a similar tape while in the bath. When the tape has finished, she begins on a series of graded finger penetration exercises, starting with the little finger inserted one knuckle at a time. There is no pressure for achievement. 'The program is given by the therapist, the pace decided by the client.'

Sessions with the couple together commence as soon as the woman begins to make some progress. Counselling focusses on the fact that both partners are concerned about the painful effects of penetration. 'Otherwise you might be here complaining of rape, not vaginismus.'

Some authorities (e.g., Munjack and Oziel[20]) suggest that the practitioner should demonstrate the insertion of a lubricated finger into the woman's vagina and then the insertion of the smallest of a series of graded dilators. The partner is invited to watch the procedure.

The advantage of this approach is that the woman leaves the practitioner's rooms with a success experience. The disadvantage may be that it further lowers the self-esteem of her partner. He has been trying to achieve penetration for some time and may perceive the practitioner's success as belittling. It can also be perceived as a very sexually charged practitioner–patient situation, and particularly when the practitioner is male may compound the situation.

We believe that, on balance, it is better to allow the woman to carry out the whole insertion process. The notion that the client is responsible for change as far as possible is one of the fundamentals of modern counselling.

INFERTILITY

Of course, infertility cannot be regarded as a sexual dysfunction as such except in special cases, such as the situation where the man suffers retarded ejaculation and fakes orgasm. However, pressure to conceive is a common concern that may cause and/or exacerbate any sexual dysfunction. Fertility is an important area of concern and one where patients need a great deal of support. This is especially so in view of the wide publicity currently given to procedures such as the *in vitro* fertilization program. Patients present with the belief that the problem can probably be fixed, and some are going to be disappointed.

The case history in Box 6-9 is rather long. We thought it worthwhile to include it because it illustrates many points relevant to infertility treatment and counselling:

- Extensive investigations were carried out.
- Time-consuming and uncomfortable procedures were involved.
- The cost of some procedures and medications was not covered by private or public health funds.
- The investigations originally focussed on one partner alone.
- Not only were the couple not offered supportive counselling, they never felt that they had been given permission to discuss sexual matters.
- The interventions and their impact on the couple's relationship appeared to be a major factor in the subsequent marriage breakdown.

How to be supportive

When a patient or couple who have been having unprotected intercourse for a year or more without a pregnancy present, take a sexual history at

---

BOX 6-9

Infertility: a case history

In early 1975, Mr and Mrs R. decided to have a family. They had been happily married for three years. He was aged 30 and she 31. She discontinued taking her (high dosage) contraceptive pill and began to take her waking temperature. The couple took care to have intercourse several times when she noted a mid-cycle temperature rise. Her cycle varied between 26 and 40 days.

After a year of trying, they consulted a gynaecologist in January 1976. He prescribed clomiphene citrate and also advised them to refrain from intercourse in the first two weeks of Mrs R.'s menstrual cycle. When she noted a rise in her waking temperature, they were to have intercourse at 18-hourly to 24-hourly intervals if possible. Mrs R. developed cycle-related mood swings, being euphoric at ovulation time and irritable or depressed premenstrually.

Mrs R. became anorgasmic with intercourse and encouraged her husband to ejaculate as soon as possible. 'It was too mechanical, not making love for two weeks and then going at it like rabbits.' In October 1976, Mrs R. had a laparoscopy, which was normal. In June 1977 Mrs R. became pregnant, but in October was diagnosed as having a hydatidiform mole. Her gynaecologist removed the mole vaginally and performed a dilation and curettage a week later. The couple were advised to use condoms or spermicide as contraception and Mrs R.'s hormone levels were monitored. After about a year, she was again prescribed clomiphene citrate.

After six clomiphene courses, the gynaecologist suggested a post-coital test. Mrs R., who attended alone, asked the nurse who carried out the test if any live sperm were present. 'No. It looks as if your vaginal fluids are killing them off.'

Mr R. was than asked to provide a semen specimen, which showed a very low sperm count. He was referred to a urologist who diagnosed a varicocele and operated.

In January 1980, Mrs R. became pregnant and delivered a full-term healthy child. Mr R. was anxious to have more children and clomiphene citrate was reinstated.

Two years later, the sexual side of the marriage had deteriorated badly. Mrs R. professed to enjoy sexual relations only when there

---

was no chance of pregnancy. Her husband found this attitude strange and disturbing.

In January 1986 the gynaecologist referred them to an endocrinologist. He ordered a hysterosalpingogram and a further laparoscopy. As Mr R.'s sperm count was again very low, he put Mrs R. on a course of Pergonal and Prophasyl. The program involved daily injections, mid-cycle daily blood scans and mid-cycle daily ultrasounds.

When she menstruated at the end of the first treatment cycle, Mrs R. declined to continue treatment. She was a solicitor and had the time-demands of a big case coming to court shortly. The recriminations that followed led up to divorce proceedings.

once. If a patient presents alone, ask to see the partner and suggest that they try to attend together whenever possible.

There are good reasons for this:

- It emphasizes that it is a shared problem. Both partners will be under similar stress.
- *Both* partners will need physical investigation and assessment. In cases where a physical cause is found, it is about 60% a female problem, 40% male.[21] A useful source on male infertility is Hellstrom's edited book.[22] Books on female infertility are more readily available, usually in the gynaecology and obstetric section of any academic medical library.
- Both partners may need counselling if problems arise. It is helpful to have an ongoing relationship with them.

Before embarking on any investigations, tell the couple honestly what they are to expect. A simple solution may be found in a short time. On the other hand the investigations and treatment procedures may be prolonged, expensive, time consuming, uncomfortable or embarrassing.

Right at the beginning, it is important to find out if both partners are equally as keen to achieve a pregnancy. Be aware that this may change, especially if interventions are focussed on one partner alone.

As far as possible, couples should be encouraged to make only minimal changes in frequency of intercourse. Even so, many people respond, as Mrs R. did, with the feeling that they have changed from a sexual person in their own right into a baby-making machine.

At all sessions, the practitioner should ask if the investigations and interventions are affecting the couple's sex life. A good preamble is, 'Some people find that this kind of treatment takes the spontaneity out of sex and makes it rather mechanical. Has that bothered either of you at all?'. If it has, you can make a cost-benefit analysis of the relative values of continuing with treatment or taking a few months off. Above all, providing couples with *permission* not to try and have fabulous sex while also trying to conceive can decrease performance pressure and decrease the chance of sexual dysfunctions developing.

Another issue to be addressed is the feeling of failure when the woman does not conceive. 'I cry every month when I see the blood on the toilet paper.' The practitioner can encourage patients to talk about this and be alert for any blaming going on in the relationship.

Of course, the fact that many couples, especially those of higher socio-economic status, are delaying starting a family until several years after marriage puts an additional stress on them when a fertility problem arises. There is the feeling that the woman's reproductive time is running out.

There are some important considerations when the treatment is deemed to be unsuccessful and terminated. If you decide to end treatment, the couple may be angry, distressed or feel abandoned. It is vital to introduce the topic of termination tentatively and perhaps be prepared to continue for a while, with a specified time limit. If the patients themselves decide to discontinue, it's very easy to feel angry yourself about the time and expertise you have invested in their case. Try to ask a non-judgmental open-ended question such as, 'What are your reasons for wanting to stop now?'. This format avoids the confrontational 'Why' and obliquely implies that they may wish to resume treatment at some future date. Partnership discord is a rather common factor in discontinuing infertility treatment. Be alert for it and be prepared to offer counselling or refer if necessary.

Finally, do not assume that the end of treatment implies the end of the couple's need for support. Many people feel a very real sense of bereavement when they have to abandon their hopes for a child and may continue to need help. In some cases, termination of treatment may represent a unilateral decision by one or other partner and be a potent source of partnership discord, as illustrated by our case history.

Linda Salzer's[23] book is a valuable source of insights into the psychological aspects of infertility. Appleton, Clark and Rainsbury[24] give further guidelines for counselling, as does Wylie.[25]

There are a wide range of interventions available in sexual counselling and treatment. Practitioners need to be knowledgeable about interventions that fall within their own range of expertise and willing to refer to specialists when something further is called for.

REFERENCES

1. Annon, J.S. *The behavioral treatment of sexual problems: brief therapy.* Honolulu: Enabling Systems, 1974.
2. Stedman, Y. The assessment of sexual dysfunction. *British Journal of Sexual Medicine,* 1994, 21: 17-19.
3. King, R. *Good loving: finding a balance when your sex drives differ: great sex.* Sydney: Random House, 1997.
4. Masters, W.H. and Johnson, V.E. *Human sexual inadequacy.* Boston: Little, Brown and Company, 1970.
5. Kaplan, H.S. *The new sex therapy.* New York: Brunner/Mazel, 1974.
6. Robinson, B.E. Whose week is it anyhow? Dealing with discrepant sexual desire in relationships. *Sexual Health Today,* 1997; 1: 1–3.
7. Coleman, E. Is your patient suffering from compulsive sexual behavior? *Psychiatric Annals,* 1992; 22(6): 320–325.
8. Kinsey, A.C., Pomeroy, W.B. and Martin, C.E. *Sexual behavior in the human male.* Philadelphia: W.B. Saunders, 1948.
9. Semans, J.H. Premature ejaculation. A new approach. *South Medical Journal,* 1956; 49: 353.
10. Wolpe, J. and Lazarus, A.A. *Behaviour therapy techniques. A guide to the treatment of neuroses.* Oxford: Pergamon Press, 1966.
11. Comfort, A. *The joy of sex. A gourmet guide.* London: Mitchell Beazley, 1987.
12. White, E. and Silverstein, C. *The joy of gay sex: an intimate guide for gay men to the pleasures of a gay lifestyle.* New York: Simon and Schuster, 1977.
13. Loulan, J. *Lesbian sex.* San Francisco: spinsters/aunt lute, 1984.
14. Loulan, J. *Lesbian passion. Loving ourselves and each other.* San Francisco: spinsters/aunt lute, 1987.
15. Kinsey, A.C., Pomeroy, W.B., Martin, C.E. and Gebhard, P.H. *Sexual behavior in the human female.* Philadelphia: W.B. Saunders, 1953.
16. Friday, N. *My Secret Garden.* New York: Pocket Books, 1973.
17. Friday, N. *Forbidden Flowers: More Women's Sexual Fantasies.* New York: Pocket Books, 1975.
18. Metz, M.E., Rosser, B.R.S. and Strapko, N. Differences in conflict-resolution styles among heterosexual, gay, and lesbian couples. *Journal of Sex Research,* 1994; 31(4): 293–308.
19. Goldberg, G. Suggestion as a general structure and a specific strategy in the behavioural treatment of vaginismus. *Australian Journal of Clinical and Experimental Hypnosis,* 1983; 11: 39–47.
20. Munjack, D.J. and Oziel, L.J. *Sexual medicine and counseling in office practice: a comprehensive treatment guide.* Boston: Little, Brown and Company, 1980.

21. Hensleigh, P. Infertility. In Barnard, M.U., Clancy, B.J. and Kramtz, K.E. (eds) *Human sexuality for health professionals*. Philadelphia: W.B. Saunders, 1978.
22. Hellstrom, W.J.S. (ed.) *Male infertility and sexual dysfunction*. New York: Springer Verlag, 1997.
23. Salzer, L. *Surviving infertility: a compassionate guide through the emotional crisis of infertility*. New York: Harper Perennial, 1991.
24. Appleton, T., Clark, M. and Rainsbury, P. *Counselling the infertile couple*. In Rainsbury, P.A. and Viniker, D.A. (eds) *Practical guide to reproductive medicine*. New York, Parthenon, 1997.
25. Wylie, K. Psychological aspects of infertility. *British Journal of Sexual Medicine*, 1994, 21: 6–9.

7 Reactions to STD infection and STD counselling

There are a number of reasons why counselling is an integral part of treating patients with STDs. First, the management of the illness, and the prevention of further infection of others or reinfection, is based on a number of behaviors that may be positively influenced by counselling. These include adherence to medication, cessation of unsafe sexual behavior and other actions likely to transmit pathogens, and alteration of current and future sexual behavior to prevent reinfection after treatment.

Second, STDs are set aside from most other conditions as being stigmatizing—indeed, even talking about sexual behavior, let alone about contracting an STD, causes difficulty for some health practitioners. In the case of widely publicized STDs, such as HIV infection and herpes, the stigmatization is sufficiently severe as to lead to overt discrimination. The degree of stigmatization may lead to psychological harm, including depression, anxiety or loss of self-esteem, as well as loss of social supports.

While important in themselves, these factors in turn are likely to influence compliance with medication and other behavioral requirements for successful treatment.

THE GOALS OF STD COUNSELLING

Counselling is a vague term which is loosely applied in health practice and is sometimes used synonymously with 'talking'. Harris and Ramsay[1] comment that counselling is never aimless talking, but rather is a clear and coherent option for defining a problem, suitable for use from the first contact with a patient. There are a number of goals specific to STD counselling.

Providing comprehensive care

The goal of counselling is for the practitioner to provide comprehensive and thorough care for the patient. It must never be a substitute for treating the illness, but rather should assist in history taking, management, compliance with treatment and prevention of future infection, as well as identification of associated psychosocial difficulties that may not have been evident initially.

Providing information

Counselling should include provision of specific information to patients which will help them to understand the condition and its management, and to prevent recurrence. This is often referred to as 'education' and should be aimed at preventing spread of disease or reinfection. This is set out in detail in chapter 11, which deals with pre- and post-test counselling.

Reducing psychological sequelae

A degree of psychological harm, usually acute but occasionally chronic, may come from the knowledge of having a socially stigmatized condition. This may range from the feeling of being 'punished' for sexual activity, to loss of self-esteem from the contraction of an unacceptable illness, to the effects of making others (such as spouse or partner) aware that their partner has had sexual contact outside a primary relationship. This latter result of an STD may itself include sequelae such as relationship breakdown, depression or anxiety, or severe or dysfunctional guilt.

Informing the partner(s)

With many STDs, it is advisable that contact tracing or partner notification, and concurrent management of partners, occur both to prevent patient reinfection and to prevent further spread of the particular disease. This sensitive area of patient management needs careful explanation as patients are often initially reluctant to contact partners. Where both partners are being simultaneously treated by the practitioner, relationship counselling may often need to occur as a function of one patient blaming the other for the STD or because the exposure of outside sexual contact leads to strains in the relationship.

THE COUNSELLING PROCESS IN STD MANAGEMENT

The counselling process can be easily followed by most health practitioners, regardless of whether they have had specific training in counselling. It requires only clear goals, a warm manner, and an understanding of the issues and processes involved. Probably the most important starting point is for the practitioner to give the patient an opportunity to express discomfort and for the practitioner to recognize this discomfort. Most patients have usually thought quite a lot about the issues before they consult a practitioner, and often have arrived at some conclusions about the nature of their problems. However, there are a number of special issues that emerge in STD and AIDS counselling which need to be addressed.

THE MEANING OF STD TO THE INDIVIDUAL

Perhaps the earliest recorded account of an STD, probably syphilis, was in China in 6237 BC,[2] yet little of a scientific nature has been written about the meaning of STD infection to the individual, and little empirical research has been carried out on this area. This chapter attempts to explain the beliefs underlying psychological reactions to STDs and the reasons for psychological problems, as well as approaches to counselling them when they occur.

In discussing the meaning of STDs to the individual, there appear to be at least five separate attributions in modern society.

1. STDs are a deserved outcome of indiscriminate sexual behavior and punishment for sexual sins.
2. STDs are a consequence of individual inadequacy that leads to sexually indiscriminate behavior.
3. STDs are a consequence of a breakdown in traditional social values and rapid social change.
4. STDs are the result of an individual coming into intimate contact with a virulent pathogen.
5. STDs are a sign of being sexually active and a matter of pride.

Note that there is a hierarchy of blame from attribution 1 to attribution 5. With the exception of attribution 5, the level of blame roughly parallels a similar hierarchy of the degree to which the individuals see themselves responsible for the infection. However, it is important to recognize that different models will apply in different cultures and subcultures, and will depend on the degree to which there is a psychological investment in sexual behavior.

Equally importantly, the meaning of STDs to the patient and to a lesser degree to the health practitioner will affect not only the compliance with treatment but also the psychological response to infection and probably the subsequent risks of exposure to STDs the patient takes. Diagnosing the psychological difficulties surrounding STDs will be made easier if the practitioner is able to assess the patient's understanding of what it means for her or him to have an STD. The practitioner can then intervene more effectively.[3]

Because the meaning of having an STD varies widely across patients, we will now focus on each category of meaning in turn. Because homosexual males are at disproportionate risk for STDs, we have chosen to focus on this population to illustrate the variety of responses and their implications for counselling.

STD as punishment

When the individual sees the STD as punishment, it is commonly the case that she or he has a particularly religious background, has never come to terms with sexuality, and has significant internalized homophobia and/or erotophobia.

In the case of homosexual men, the individual will probably be at one of the first three stages of homosexual adjustment described by Cass,[4] in which their sexual orientation is not usually publicly acknowledged and almost invariably not accepted. Cass's stages are (1) identity confusion; (2) identity comparison; (3) identity tolerance; (4) identity acceptance; (5) identity pride; and (6) identity synthesis (these stages are discussed in more detail in chapter 13).

The combination of the stigma of STD with the stigma of homosexuality is an extremely powerful one, and the homosexual STD patient who sees his infection as an indication that he is being punished will need careful attention. The result of infection is likely to include remorse about his sexuality, which in turn increases his internalized homophobia. Clinical or subclinical depression ensues as the individual is faced with the evidence of a sexual behavior that he has probably compartmentalized or denied. This applies equally well to heterosexual people who have not accepted that sexual behavior has occurred, or that it has occurred outside a primary relationship. There may also be anxiety about discovery or exposure. In such cases the anxiety or embarrassment may lead to defaulting from treatment, denial of a homosexual orientation (or heterosexual contact outside a primary relationship) in the first place, and commitment to never be (homo) sexual again.

Ross[5] has noted that a significant percentage of STD clinic attenders who are homosexual deny their sexual orientation to the attending practitioner, and that these individuals are most likely to expect the most negative reactions to their sexuality from others. Such individuals who deny homosexual or extramarital contact are also most likely to be first attenders, and those who attend private practitioners rather than public clinics may tend to deny their sexuality to a greater extent. It is important that the practitioner does not accept or reinforce the patient's negative view of his sexuality, particularly as this may be one of the first times the patient has admitted his sexual orientation or contacts to anyone outside a small circle. Reinforcing homophobia is inappropriate for two reasons: first, for the individual, where the homophobia is severe, significant suicidality may also be present. By reinforcing homophobia, you risk causing significant harm. Second, homophobia is not a successful long-term deterrent preventing homosexual activity. Rosser and colleagues[6] have recently demonstrated that, of men who have sex with other men, those with highest levels of internalized homophobia while they may try to avoid homosexual activity, are 7 to 12 times less likely to use condoms when they do engage in sex.

Sometimes patients who have in the past apparently accepted their sexuality return to the first and most negative attribution of blame when they contract one of the more severe STDs. As an example, some people with AIDS or herpes who have been living openly homosexual (or 'fast lane' heterosexual) lives have seen their disease as a 'punishment from God' and blamed it on their sexuality. In some cases this may also be associated with an increase in religiosity in a person with AIDS. The combination of sexuality and STDs is a psychologically powerful one: for the patient's mental well-being, if it is apparent that they see their STD infection as a 'punishment', assessment of the need for reassurance or correction must be made. The situation is more difficult if this is part of the patient's 'acceptance' of AIDS and/or death. In such cases, it is helpful to have access to accepting clergy for referral.

Venereophobias and the 'worried well'

The first category of the meaning of infection to the individual, the notion of an STD as a punishment, is most notable for its mental health consequences, which in many cases require more attention than the STD. Venereophobia, in which there is no evidence of STD infection but where the patient is convinced that infection has occurred, most commonly occurs in patients who see it as punishment for some real or imagined misdeed, usually of a sexual nature (see Box 7-1). The attention given to HIV infection and AIDS in the past few years has made 'AIDS phobias' a reasonably common clinical phenomenon. The individuals presenting with the phobia are usually concerned over sexual contact outside primary relationships, and

BOX 7-1
AIDS phobia

Mr C., a 25-year-old waiter, presented on referral from a hospital physician. He had been convinced he had AIDS for the past three weeks. He had been living in a heterosexual relationship for the past four years, and his partner had become pregnant three months previously. The sole risk factors for HIV infection were two homosexual encounters (both insertor fellatio) in the past year, one in Australia and one in southern Europe. He had subsequently avoided any further homosexual enounters from fear of contracting AIDS.

Symptoms on presentation included mild unilateral cervical lymphadenopathy, arthralgia, fatigue and insomnia, and suicidal ideation associated with the thought that he was going to die of AIDS.

Mr C. had had hepatitis A one year previously and had convinced himself this was cancer; three years previously he had convinced himself he had herpes following another homosexual encounter. Apart from severe psoriasis from the age of 17, there was no history of medical or psychiatric illness.

Mr C.'s attitudes to homosexuality were negative: he stated that he had no emotional attraction to males, had homosexual encounters only for the physical pleasure, and was as hurtful as possible in rejecting those who had fellated him. As an adolescent he had actively encouraged his peers to attack homosexual men, and he now saw AIDS as 'God's judgement on homosexuals'.

Four weeks previously, Mr C. had completed a course of hypnotherapy, in which he had talked about his homosexual activities and his guilt over them for the first time, and been advised that there was no reason to punish himself over this. On presentation his DSM axis I diagnosis was hypochondriasis, and his belief that he had AIDS was of delusional quality.

Two sessions of interpretive psychotherapy and a negative confirmatory HIV antibody test result (which Mr C. would not initially believe) enabled him to see the relationship between his previous beliefs that he had cancer or herpes and his present belief he had AIDS. His insight into the dynamics of his disease conviction suggested it was delusional as initially suspected. He was also able to recognize that the surfacing of the issue of his homosexual behavior during hypnotherapy had apparently forced his denial of his bisexuality towards affective discharge, and the subsequent decompensation had resulted in his belief that he had AIDS as a 'punishment'. A further contributor was the ambivalence he felt over his partner's pregnancy and his uncertainty over marriage and settling down. On follow-up three months later, Mr C. admitted to still occasionally thinking about AIDS but these thoughts were not intrusive and he was trying to avoid homosexual encounters to reduce dissonance between his sexual attitudes and activities. His arthralgia and fatigue had been further investigated and a diagnosis of rheumatoid arthritis was subsequently made.

are experiencing stress at work or in relationships which often acts as a trigger. Ross[7] has suggested that when such patients are provided with insight into the additional factors that have led them to present with their concern at this time, the issue of HIV infection will often drop away and the other concerns (guilt over sexual behavior or outside sexual relationships for which the possibility of HIV infection is 'punishment') will emerge.

Brief insight-oriented counselling is the treatment of choice provided there is no evidence of psychosis. It is important not to perform repeated HIV testing, which may only reinforce the patient's conviction of infection. Paradoxical interventions[8] have been suggested as appropriate to psychotherapy for people with intractable AIDS worry, but these interventions (which involve treating individuals as if they were infected in order to release them from their rigid and distressing beliefs) should be carried out only by competent psychotherapists.

STDs as evidence of maladjustment

This second category of meaning has much in common with the first category in which STDs are seen as a punishment. While the reason for the individual's dysphoria on realizing that he or she has an STD may be a result of lack of acceptance of his or her sexual orientation, the basis is not religious and the discomfort not so pronounced. Although the major difficulties are also likely to be psychological, denial through keeping sexual orientation separate from other aspects of life may also be present. Married men frequently fall into this category, and their homosexual activities are thus more likely to be anonymous (e.g., to occur in public restrooms), which enables physical contact to occur while emotional contact is avoided. (Humphreys[9] found that over half of the men who had sex in public toilets were married.) As a result, the contacts are often likely to be unknown, and there is the added complication that the patient's wife may have been infected and be unaware of her spouse's bisexuality. Since a sizeable proportion of homosexual men (between 10% and 20%) marry, and since those who marry are usually those less accepting of their homosexuality,[10] such people may have significant internalized homophobia. A comparable situation will occur in the case of the person who has had extramarital contact.

In contrast to situations where individuals are unhappy at being homosexual (or at having affairs outside a primary relationship or frequent sexual contacts), patients in this second category become disturbed by their sexuality only when it produces negative consequences such as STD infection. The advent of AIDS has also produced a marked increase in patients falling into this category in the past few years.

A second group within this category are those with mild discomfort who have a treatable STD infection, and who recognize that there is nothing they can do about their sexual behavior but feel that it might be easier to be monogamous (or heterosexual). They rarely present a problem in terms of either compliance with treatment or of mental state. On the other hand, too great a degree of discomfort may result in sexual contacts that are anonymous, because for some people known partners and emotional contact could be too guilt-engendering. Contact tracing is thus likely to be difficult, although having the patient return for proof of cure is usually not a problem. Treatment of this attributional group is similar to that of the first group if 'AIDS phobias' arise, and may require psychotherapy.

STDs as the fault of a sick society

In this group, the blame for STD infection is likely to be projected towards others rather than internalized, and the individual, if homosexual, is most likely to be at Cass's[4] fifth stage of homosexual development. The fifth stage, according to Cass, is the period where the individual accepts his homosexuality and defines his whole lifestyle in terms of it. Thus, when he allocates blame for STD infection, it cannot lie with his sexual orientation, which is so centrally important to him, but must lie elsewhere. Elsewhere is usually the society that so stigmatizes homosexual people that it may be necessary (although much less so than in the past) to meet in secluded places and keep sexual contacts concealed.

Stigmatization may also affect the number of sexual partners by lowering a person's self-esteem to the point where relationships are not possible, and either multiple partners or no partners may be the adjustment sought to counter a negative self-image. While these arguments are based on reality in places where sexuality is severely stigmatized and legal penalties are also severe, or in rural areas or small towns, they appear seldom to apply to those whose sexuality (particularly homosexuality and/or masculinity) is the central defining construct of their lifestyle. Essentially, those who believe that STDs are the fault of a discriminatory society are unable to accept that any fault lies with them, and may be less responsive to suggestions about cutting down at-risk practices. In some cases, such a suggestion will be construed as a condemnation of their sexuality, and the consultation terminated. In others, STD infection becomes a matter of pride, indicating emancipation from the perceived restrictive and conservative sexual habits of monogamy and 'ownership' of sexual partners. Where sexual behavior is seen as a political or social statement, it is less likely that it will be open to modification.

Similarly, where an individual has recently 'come out' as homosexual or become heterosexually active, it is most likely that there will be more frequent sexual contacts. This increase in sexual contacts occurs in response to a previous lack of sexual contact in most cases; and because the person needs to develop psychosexually and is in Coleman's[11] stage of experimentation (Coleman's stages are discussed in more detail in chapter 13). Sexual activity in these cases may also be higher than it would otherwise be due to an affirmation of the individual's core identity—as public understanding of homosexuality and heterosexuality centres on their sexual component rather than their emotional or social component. If this is the case, then suggestions that attempt to modify sexual behavior could be seen as a rejection of a person's sexuality, and thus the point should be approached cautiously. If, however, this does not appear to be occurring after a lapse of several years, it may be advisable to raise the issue by determining the meaning of sexual behavior to the patient and by attempting to identify any personal difficulties that may be driving their sexual behavior. Generally, patients at this stage represent the opposite of the 'STD as punishment' group, in that the latter see their sexuality as inviting retribution while the former see their sexuality as a central, defining and positive aspect of their lifestyle.

STDs as just another infection

For some people, STD infection is not highly emotionally laden and carries no investment. Such individuals are likely, if homosexual, to be in Cass's stage 5 or stage 6, in which a homosexual orientation is seen as being only one of many identifications the individual has, and not central to identity or lifestyle. Of course, many STD infections (HIV and herpes excepted) are medically curable, with varying risks associated, but few people are able to see it that way. In terms of dealing with individuals at this stage of STD perception, there is little problem in making suggestions of modification of at-risk behaviors; but, on the other hand, if infection does not cause psychological distress there is little reason to do so unless the risk is a major one and incurable (such as with hepatitis B or C, or HIV) or the effects are long term (such as herpes).

People who have this attribution of the cause of STDs tend to have identified themselves as actively heterosexual, bisexual or homosexual for a longer period and approach sexuality in a fairly hedonistic way. Thus, if modification to partner numbers as a response to AIDS or other STDs is necessary, partner numbers may be cut down without great psychological trauma. However, if partner numbers are important to the person's self-esteem, then that individual may externalize the blame and see STDs as the 'fault of a sick society'.

STDs as a source of pride

In some situations, cultures and subcultures, particularly for male adolescents who are eager to demonstrate their maturity by demonstrating sexual conquest or desirability, STDs may be a source of pride, rite of entry or badge of masculinity. In such a situation, it will be difficult to suggest preventive measures since they may diminish the individual's identity as adult or sexually desirable and threaten one of his sources of self-esteem. Such individuals may also fall into the fifth stage—'identity pride'—of Cass's model, and may see attempts to reduce the chances of reoccurrence (although not cure of individual episodes) as diminishing what may be perceived as a mark of prestige among peers. With the advent of AIDS, however, this attitude has become less common. It may be possible to invest condom use with some of the positive properties of STDs in this attribution as a preventive strategy.

STD COUNSELLING

As in other areas of counselling, the goals of STD counselling should be clear. They include:

- To help the patient or client to have a realistic understanding of their disease

- To educate the patient about necessary treatment
- To prevent future occurrences of other STDs for the patient
- To prevent transmission of the disease to others.

Realistic understanding

Given the meanings of STDs discussed above, it is important to start by understanding what having an STD means to the patient. In counselling, the aim should be to assist the patient to gain a realistic understanding: not so pathologized that the patient suffers significant psychological harm, nor so trivialized that the patient dismisses the infection as unimportant. In most cases, the patient is likely to overpathologize; hence it is important to balance this tendency with reassuring information. In some cases, particularly where the person feared the symptoms were those of HIV, diagnosis with a (non-HIV) STD may actually be relieving to the patient. Therefore, it is important to ask the patient how he or she feels following diagnosis. Providing written, easy-to-understand information on the particular STD is important. Normalizing feelings of guilt and shame as transient reactions following an STD can also be helpful.

For STDs that are likely to be recurrent (e.g., herpes), the practitioner should spend time reviewing what signs and symptoms a patient should note, and what this means for infectivity. In particular, patients need specific direction on when they can resume sexual activity. Assistance should be given in understanding asymptomatic recurrences, infectiousness to others, and what behavioral modification is necessary.

Treatment education

Obviously, this will vary according to the specific STD(s) diagnosed. Particularly in cross-cultural settings and settings where language is a barrier, it is important to ensure instructions are clearly understood. When providing oral medication, for example, ensure that the patient knows to take the medication orally, not as a suppository. Asking the patient to repeat back to you any medication instructions can clarify the patient's understanding.

Preventing future occurrences

Any diagnosis with an STD is a natural opportunity to discuss prevention. However, STD prevention education varies widely from highly effective interventions to useless imparting of information that leaves the patient confused and feeling abandoned. The following principles are important for effective prevention:

- Individualize prevention education. Just providing a pamphlet or launching into condom use 101 is insufficient for most people to modify their behavior, although written materials should certainly be provided as background and back-up information.
- Help the patient to identify risk factors and co-factors: When are you most at risk for engaging in unsafe sex? What things make it more likely for you not to use a condom?
- Focus on behavior *patterns*. While many patients may prefer to see an STD as a 'freak' occurrence, most STDs occur following a pattern of risk behavior.
- Work with the patient to develop an individualized plan to prevent further STDs. For example, if a patient is more likely to engage in unprotected sex when feeling depressed, ask the person to identify early signs of depression for her or him, and then work together on solving the problem. What specific situations for the future are of most concern?
- In developing an individual plan, keep in mind that small changes in behavior are more manageable and successful than total lifestyle changes.
- Just telling a patient to use condoms is not sufficient. If patients report a dislike of using condoms, work with them to identify the reasons they don't use them, then develop a realistic plan for introducing condom use into future sexual activity. For example, if a man complains that he has decreased sensitivity when using condoms, you can suggest putting some lubricant inside the tip, or using the 'female' condom. A couple who didn't use condoms because they were 'in love' can be encouraged to examine the idea that part of loving is looking after one's own and one's partner's health. The man who fears erectile failure or inability to ejaculate when using condoms can be assisted by reframing the problem to focus specifically on these concerns.
- While most sexually active patients have experimented with condoms at least once, some patients may report never having used condoms. In these cases, demonstrating condom use in the practitioner's office is most effective. In particular, having the patient handle the condom and practise putting it on by demonstrating on two of your fingers increases the chance of future use. Box 7-2 outlines the important points to cover when demonstrating condoms to patients.
- Consider referral for follow-up counselling as appropriate. A helpful insight is to view risk behavior both as a problem in itself and as possibly symptomatic of other underlying concerns. Studies in HIV prevention have identified many co-factors of risk including concurrent drug/alcohol, depression and other mental health concerns; sexual anxiety; history of abuse; lack of assertiveness; sexual orientation dis-

---

BOX 7-2

Demonstrating condom use to patients

The following facts are the most important when introducing condoms to patients:

- First, condoms should be kept close by for any encounter. Does the patient keep condoms in the bedroom or carry them when going out?
- Second, condoms have a shelf life (two to three years) and should be stored in a reasonably cool place. When opening condoms, the patient should take care not to rip the condom.
- Third, lubricant helps. Keep water-based lubricant for use in condoms with the condoms. A little inside the tip adds sensitivity.
- Fourth, roll the condom on the right way. (The unrolled condom should have the teat at the top). Rolled on the right way it should slide down the fingers (penile shaft).
- Fifth, some masturbation in maintaining the erection may be required. This is entirely normal.
- Sixth, when withdrawing hold on to the condom.
- It's a good idea for men who haven't used condoms before to practise by putting one on when masturbating alone. Practice builds familiarity and confidence in using condoms, so providing condoms for the patient to practise with is recommended.
- It is also important to check whether the patient has sufficient assertiveness to buy condoms, and to ask whether there are any other barriers to use.

---

tress; patterns of compulsive sexual behavior; and internalized homophobia. These should be viewed as serious medical concerns necessitating referral as appropriate. Chapter 4 provided screening questions and surveys to assist the patient and practitioner to identify common reasons for risk behavior.

Preventing disease transmission to others

Depending on the STD, many clients have additional questions on how to tell current or future partners about their STD. The stress of disclosure should not be underestimated. For example, a patient treated by one of the authors (SR) was a highly successful and senior judge, yet avoided intimate relationships for many years because she contracted genital herpes. In her country, and certainly by those who came before her, she was viewed as highly assertive, successful and powerful, yet she carried deep shame for what she considered her terrible secret. In addition to issues of partner notification, it is important to discuss, and if necessary ask to role-play, how the person will disclose this information in future situations.

Without summarizing in detail the many issues that STD infection may elicit or precipitate, it is important to note two points. First, the practitioner will probably be the only individual with whom the patient will be able to discuss the infection (and thus fulfils an important role as a supportive listener for a wide range of conflicts and concerns). Second, as already noted, the stigmatization surrounding STDs may precipitate a number of dysphoric mood states, or identity or relationship crises, which require just as much in the way of identification and management as will the infection itself.

PRACTITIONER REACTIONS TO STDS

Patients are not the only ones with beliefs about STDs: the five meanings of STDs described above are just as applicable for practitioners. Those who have read widely on the subject will be able to classify various authors and authorities on a continuum from seeing gonococci as 'God's little helpers' through to approaching them as just a part of infectious disease management. The important thing to note is that our attitudes as practitioners will affect our approach to our patients, and that our personal attitudes will interact with those of our patients. The consequence of this for modification of risky behaviors is enormous, as shown in the following two examples. On the one hand, the practitioner whose attribution of STDs is as a punishment from God will discourage avoidance of risks because the 'punishment' is preordained and presumably unavoidable. Nor will any distinction be made between safe and unsafe sexual acts because the 'punishment' is seen as being for sexual activity, not specific sexual acts! On the other hand, the practitioner who believes that sexuality is important and that STDs are just another infection may have less motivation to encourage individuals to modify their behaviors. Either extreme is unhelpful. Where practitioners see sexual contact in ideological terms—either as punishment or as licence—the practitioners need to address their own values and attitudes. Otherwise, the interaction between patients and practitioners who hold conflicting attributions for STDs may also lead to tension, anger, transference and counter-transference issues, and to resistance to taking advice or to treatment, particularly where more divergent attributions are held. It is critical to ascertain your own position and make some estimate of the position of your patient before trying to educate, or to modify risky behaviors.

Two exercises can be helpful here. First, to increases self-awareness, ask yourself how you really feel about STDs. How would you—or how did you—feel having an STD yourself? Write down your own values and attitudes. Second, to examine how your attitudes may affect patients, write down the logical consequences for a practitioner of having these attitudes. In particular, list both the positive and negative consequences for your patients of having you as their practitioner!

GENITAL HERPES INFECTIONS AND COUNSELLING

Herpes simplex infection of the genital region falls midway in its implications and impact between the essentially curable bacterial STDs and HIV. While herpes is not a fatal infection there is no cure, although treatment for *individual episodes* is available. However, counselling those with herpes is particularly important because there has been some suggestion that recurrent viral infection may be influenced by psychological factors.

Linking psychological status and recurrence

The recurrence of herpes simplex virus (HSV) disease has been linked with both psychological and physiological factors.

Drob and colleagues[12] noted that lack of social skills, including *assertiveness*, and inability to vent emotions may be associated with recurrences, and Goldmeir[13] has linked non-psychotic psychological *states*, such as anxiety and *obsessiveness*, to high frequencies of recurrence. Psychotherapy was shown to reduce frequency of herpes episodes, and over three quarters of people with HSV regarded stress as a major factor in their recurrence. Further, the stress of having HSV was felt to prime new recurrences. Thus it is important both to note that there may be a link between psychological state and recurrence, and to attempt to break that nexus or to reduce the stressors.

Effects on lifestyle

The impact of HSV infection upon significant life areas should not be underestimated. Drob and colleagues[12] found that the majority of people

101

with genital HSV reported that infection and concern about recurrence made them less capable of physical warmth and intimacy; they enjoyed sex less, and felt less sexually desirable. All the patients in Drob's study found that work performance was hampered. It is important to ascertain the specific effects of the infection (or concern about the infection) on significant life areas and to acknowledge these as a possible focus for intervention. In the same study, a majority of those surveyed reported disturbance of affect (feeling that herpes is incompatible with happiness, and being pessimistic about the future course of the illness), and Drob and colleagues also note that in an earlier survey conducted by the American Social Health Association, 84% of people with genital herpes also reported depression.

Sexual dysfunction

Both studies reported above found that genital herpes infection had sexual consequences. Such consequences included reduced interest in sex, lowered ability to achieve orgasm, avoidance of intimacy, and less enjoyment of sex when it did occur. This is probably associated with feeling less sexually desirable because of herpes (reported by over two thirds of respondents), and feeling repugnant to others.

Providing psychological support

Interpersonal relations may also be affected by the infection or, more frequently, by concern about its effect on relationships if it is generally known that the person is infected. Aral and colleagues[14] report that over 30% of Americans say that they would not associate with someone who has herpes, and Drob and colleagues[12] also noted that the majority of their patients felt they would not be accepted by others if their herpes infection became known. In the same study, the lack of social support from others in dealing with herpes was also seen as a major problem, as was being prevented from getting to know people to whom one is sexually attracted. In this sort of situation, it is important that the practitioner be prepared to provide psychological support as well as professional advice.

Managing altered affect

Affect may also be altered by infection—the degree to which this may be physical ('post-viral depression') or psychological is not known. Nevertheless, the alteration may be sufficiently profound to consider anxiolytic or antidepressant medication in some cases. The most common concerns expressed by those with HSV infection include concern about infecting others, recurrence and the future course of the illness, and sometimes self-destructive feelings.

These general guidelines for counselling are based on the situation of chronic recurrent viral infections such as herpes, but generally apply to similar infections. There are more similarities than differences between herpes and recently diagnosed HIV infection, and what is true about herpes will also be true for HIV (and vice versa)—although reactions to herpes will generally be less severe than reactions to HIV. Nevertheless, experience in the psychological responses of people with herpes and counselling of those affected have tended to focus on heterosexual individuals, while to date the HIV literature has focussed on homosexual men.

STAGING OF REACTIONS TO HIV AND AIDS

The emotional impact of HIV infection appears to be qualitatively and quantitatively different from that of curable STDs.[15] A diagnosis of herpes may be assumed to have a similar, if lesser, impact, given that the disease is incurable, if not life-threatening.

There are stages of response to the diagnosis through which individuals may pass. In many ways, these stages are similar to those described by Elizabeth Kübler-Ross[16] in her description of patterns seen when a person is coming to terms with a diagnosis of terminal illness. They do, however, differ in some important respects since the trauma may include stigmatization as well as the possibility of death.

It is important to note that the emotional impact of a diagnosis of HIV infection is not significantly different from that of a diagnosis of full-blown AIDS. Rosser and Ross[15] found that the emotional distress of receiving a positive HIV antibody test was not significantly different from that caused by a diagnosis of AIDS, symptomatic HIV, a diagnosis of AIDS in a lover or the death of a lover, even though they appreciated that the changes in lifestyle necessitated by the events varied considerably. Their sample also reported greater perceived stress in response to negative life events than did an uninfected comparison group.

Ross, Tebble and Viliunas[17] have described the reactions of homosexual men to asymptomatic HIV infection, summarized later. They note that HIV infection may not lead to death, and hence the Kübler-Ross model of response to a terminal diagnosis may not always be appropriate.

The stages bear some similarities to models of homosexual identity formation. This is to be expected. Firstly, there is considerable stigma attached to infection with HIV or herpes and the stigmatized status is not usually visible or identifiable. Secondly, a significant proportion of individuals carrying antibodies to HIV in the western world are homosexual or bisexual men. In many cases they will use a previously appropriate and successful coping strategy to manage a second stigmatized status.

The authors note that individuals may show retrogression as well as progression between stages: some individuals may neither experience every stage nor go beyond a certain point.

It might also be of value for the practitioner to be aware that in close-knit relationships, the patient's partner may pass through these stages in parallel with him or her.

Stages 1 and 2: Shock, denial and anger

The initial stages describe the common reactions to major unanticipated trauma.

Denial may operate as a defence to prevent decompensation. The psychological processes operating commonly include guilt at being responsible for infection, and powerlessness associated with lack of control or knowledge of outcome. This may be exacerbated by associated minority status (further stigmatization within and beyond an already stigmatized group).

Helpful responses by the health practitioner are to be quietly supportive and to allow the person to progress at his or her own rate.

During the early phases, the person cannot take in much information; therefore it is appropriate to avoid overload. It is also usually unhelpful to encourage patients to express their emotions. Take your cues from the patient.

At this point it can be a good thing to review with the patient a plan of action between this initial session and follow-up (ideally 48–72 hours following diagnosis).

Stage 3: Withdrawal

This stage describes the response to recognition that one has an infection. This recognition may lead to isolation, either imposed or self-imposed, sexual or social. Recognition of the stigma associated with infection may activate previously successful coping strategies in groups such as homosexuals and injecting drug users.

Individuals at this stage tend to keep to themselves as part of their uncertainty about the reactions of others. Other salient factors in the withdrawal may be related to fear of infecting others and to depression.

One of the reasons why a follow-up appointment after diagnosis is appropriate is that it allows you to monitor how withdrawn the patient has become.

The roles of the practitioner during this phase include monitoring the patient's isolation (and in some circumstances, suicidal ideation) and being a confidante of the patient.

Stage 4: Bargaining

Substage 4A: 'Coming out' to significant others

Stage 4 is similar to a level of homosexual identity formation. The individual who is positive for HIV antibodies or herpes infection typically discloses the situation to those who are most likely to be accepting, family or significant others.

Psychological processes may include negotiating the need for acceptance, expressing the need still to be loved and displacing stress onto people taken into confidence.

The form the reactions of others take may contribute to problems relating to the stress of the disclosure itself as well as to issues of rejection and confrontation.

The health practitioner's role during this phase includes being a resource for the patient, their family and their significant others.

For the newly diagnosed person, the practitioner can assist by being a safe person for discussing how to disclose infectious status and to whom. Wherever possible, it is helpful for the practitioner to gently place the question of whom to tell back on the patient, discussing the pros and cons of disclosure in each individual case. As the patient tells others, he or she may have specific questions about HIV or herpes, safety from infection and so forth. Others may need help processing their emotional reactions.

Substage 4B: Looking for others

Here the patient seeks out other people in a similar situation, looking for the social and psychological support of those with a similar diagnosis. Sharing problems and reactions with those 'in the same boat' is a potent source of information, comfort and coping strategies.

Difficulties that may emerge include dependence on similarly infected peers, disease status becoming the dominant source of identity, and loss of anonymity when the patient becomes publicly a member of a particular group.

Previously the practitioners role may have been a rather dominant one, journeying with the patient during his or her adjustment. Now the primary role is to facilitate meetings with supportive similar others.

Substage 4C: Special status

Substage 4C turns alienation into an advantage, where individuals see themselves as different and special, needed by others.

Psychologically, this stage may represent reaction formation to a sense of guilt or self-blame for becoming infected, leading to action in substage 4D.

Problems associated with this stage include overidentification with and dependency on one's 'special' status, and splitting the world into an 'us and them' dichotomy. Self-help groups may foster this as a stage towards acceptance.

During this phase, conflicts may emerge between practitioner and patient as the patient questions the practitioner's competence. The practitioner's role now includes affirming the patient's developmental process: that for someone in this stage, his or her disease may be all-consuming.

Patients who have had no ambivalence about a previously stigmatized status such as homosexual orientation often move directly to substage 4D, omitting this stage.

Substage 4D: Altruistic behavior

Altruistic behavior connects the issues in 4B and 4C and puts them into action. There is a feeling of community and belonging to be found within the infected subgroup. The desire to help others in a similar situation may be part of the process of 'making friends with one's disease'.

The need to be of service to others may lead to burn-out and overreaction. This is balanced by the fact that it gives purpose in a life disrupted by the diagnosis and serves as a coping mechanism.

It is important ethically for the practitioner not to manipulate people in this stage to serve the greater good. Where a patient wishes to 'go public' or to leave their job to work full time helping others, the primary role of the practitioner is to assist the person to make such decisions in freedom, to explore motivations and, as with all health concerns, to assist the patient to make decisions that are healthy and realistic.

Stage 5: Acceptance

The acceptance of a perceived negative status is to be regarded as a resolution of the conflict engendered by the initial diagnosis. Integration of herpes infection or positive HIV status as part of the patient's identity occurs. This appears to be a balance between the altruism of substage 4D and attention to self.

Problems that tend to present are resistance to further change of those behaviors that may place self or others at risk, and a degree of apathy over health status.

Of course, many patients will simply not reach this stage.

Overall implications

HIV in many ways is revolutionizing the way we conduct health care.

While no one strategy is appropriate for everyone, for healthy long-term adjustment a patient-empowerment approach is usually recommended. Such an approach views health practitioners as important consultants—part of a team led by an informed patient who is the manager of his or her health. For health practitioners and patients who use such a style, the practitioner–patient relationship is often experienced as extraordinary, powerful, and as part of the best tradition of health care.

Here, authoritarian, unilateral decision-making by practitioners is inappropriate and potentially harmful. The patient's perceptions of co-operation and care are paramount (see Box 7-3)

Sexual patterns following diagnosis

Along with the psychological stages of reaction to diagnosis, it is important to note that any diagnosis of illness also has sexual sequelae.

BOX 7-3

Patient responses to perceived inappropriate reactions of carers

One of the authors (SR) has watched several patients with HIV/AIDS refuse to be attended by nurses and even specialist consultants because they refused to take their cue from the patient.

One patient who was threatening to sue the hospital if the top consultant entered his room explained: 'I can see him if and when I get better. I'm simply too ill to have to be educating the homophobic doctor arsehole today. I need to focus on my health'.

Another hospitalized patient called his primary doctor after a nurse mentioned that she felt terrible because he looked so sick. 'Get her out of here. She means well, but her energy is so negative. I don't need it. I want to get better. I want to live.'

While the sexual patterns are less well documented and defined, several patterns exist.

For many, possibly most, patients, as they go through the first stage of shock, denial and anger they experience a loss of libido and even sexual functioning. They describe their sexual desire as having left them.

During withdrawal, many patients may not be sexual with others, but may begin through masturbation to adjust sexually. Some men and women describe relating to their semen and vaginal fluids in a new way, seeing them as dirty and dangerous, symbolic of the disease that infected them.

During the fourth stage, sexual behavior with one's partner—or for singles typically safer sex, often with other HIV positives—resumes.

During the fifth stage, the person's sexuality and sexual behavior patterns start to return to the levels existing prior to diagnosis, with the exception that safer sex for most people takes on a new importance.

It is helpful for practitioners to view sexual activity as part of a person's wider process, including coping with stress. Whether through solo masturbation, sex with a significant other, or casual sexual activity, many people find sex to be powerfully releasing, distracting, grounding, affirming and/or reassuring. People undergoing profound stress, including the newly diagnosed, may also use sex to cope (both functionally and dysfunctionally).

A small minority of newly diagnosed persons with HIV may binge sexually following diagnosis. While some authors have suggested that this is an angry retribution reaction, in our experience it occurs primarily in persons with a history of compulsive sexual behavior and may more accurately and simply be defined as a person relapsing into previous behavioral patterns. When testing for HIV, asking patients how they have coped with previous stressors and taking a good sexual history will clearly be helpful, as these may predict and prevent such behavior.

It is important to address unsafe sex patterns, particularly with persons living with HIV. Rather than giving advice—'You must always practise safer sex'—it is more helpful for the health professional to establish a relationship where both practitioner and patient can raise safer-sex concerns.

Rosser, Gobby and Carr[18] in a recent study of 106 HIV positive persons found that one in four HIV positive persons admitted having unprotected sex with HIV negative or HIV status unknown persons post-diagnosis, and 10% believed they had infected others post-diagnosis. HIV positive persons having unsafe sex did not differ from positives who mantained safer sex—both knew the rules and had experience with safer sex. Hence, providing safer-sex education is not sufficient; you must specifically address the unsafe sex. The goal of such counselling should be to promote the sexual health of the patient: first, by assisting the client to recognize his or her risk behavior patterns, antecedents and co-factors; and second, by addressing these patterns through treatment and referral (see the section on the goals of STD counselling above).

Abnormal illness behaviors in STDs

Few data are available on illness behavior in STDs: it was generally assumed that illness behaviors in STDs were identical to those in other comparable illnesses. However, illness behavior has important implications for treatment. In the case of individuals with an erroneous conviction that they have an STD, which Hart[19] refers to as venereoneurosis, there is abnormal illness behavior in terms of both general hypochondriasis and a strong disease conviction without demonstrable evidence of infection. There may also be an indication that the patient believes they 'deserve' the infection. The reaction of other individuals—which is perhaps more commonly found—is a refusal to see STD as an illness; rather, it may be regarded only as a minor non-significant risk of a particular lifestyle.

Clinical observation has tended to suggest that in the case of the absence of illness behavior, patients may frequently compromise treatment: by discontinuing medication after symptoms have resolved; by continuing sexual activity after symptom resolution but before clearance; or by not returning for proof of cure. Thus, both abnormal illness behavior and lack of illness behavior may have implications for the management of STDs.

Ross[20] looked at illness behaviors in STD clinic attenders, and found that contrary to expectations, it was the repeating attenders rather than the first attenders who displayed the greatest anxiety and hypochondriasis over STD infection. Those with higher previous numbers of infections also tended to deny life stresses more, and to attribute their problems to the episode of illness. Such individuals also displayed symptom preoccupation, and higher levels of symptom exaggeration. In comparison, first attenders tended to deny that an STD was an illness, which would appear to be in some cases also a denial of the contraction of an often stigmatizing illness. Compared with other illness behaviors, in which there may be substantial secondary gain from sympathy and assistance, STD infection appears to be quite different and to develop as a function of repeated infections. In such cases, it would appear that STD infection tends to be seen as a chance event until several infections have occurred, when it is then seen not only as an illness but also as a result of particular behaviors.

In the same study, Ross also found that for STD infections there were few differences in illness behavior between heterosexual and homosexual men, apart from the fact that there is a less negative reaction to STD infection in the gay community (probably as a result of the greater awareness of STDs in gay subcultures and the greater self-definition of homosexual men in sexual terms). It was also noted, using non-STD controls attending general practice and psychiatric outpatient clinics, that the STD clinic population was closer to the psychiatric population than the general practice one. This tends to confirm the finding of Catalan and colleagues[21] that 40% of a United Kingdom STD clinic population had some degree of psychological disturbance on a screening test. It is unclear whether the disturbance was a function of having a stigmatized illness such as an STD or inherent in STD clinic attenders. There may be major differences between public and private clinics, and between the accuracy of admissions at STD clinics, depending on individual factors such as practitioner approach and clinic environment.

ADMISSION OF DETAILS OF SEXUALITY

The picture that emerges of the variables predictive of whether the patient reveals a homosexual orientation (and, one might assume, other details about his or her sexuality) when presenting to an STD clinic or health practitioner is a coherent one. Non-admitters are likely to conceal their sexuality or homosexuality from most people, to expect the most negative social reaction to their sexuality or homosexuality from significant others and society in general, and to believe in much more rigid and conservative behaviors as being appropriate for men and women. As compared with those who admit to homosexual contact, non-admitters are also more likely to report themselves as having had no previous STDs. The non-admitter thus emerges as an individual who expects particularly negative reactions to revealing his or her sexuality.

These data have a number of practical applications for counselling. A lack of previous sexually transmitted infections in non-admitters suggests that the clinic situation will be a new and potentially frightening one, in which condemnation is expected; in subsequent visits to a clinic the patient will tend to be less apprehensive if the clinician's approach has been nonjudgmental. Thus, the first visit is crucial in building up the rapport that is so critical for taking sexual histories and for sexual counselling. The apparent passivity and lack of assertion that are also predictors of failure to reveal matters about one's sexuality, suggest that many patients may have trouble expressing what is construed as negative information that may elicit a negative response. It may also be that when clinicians take histories in a manner that implies any sexual contact was a heterosexual or homosexual one, the patient may not have the courage to make a correction.

However, these psychological factors will clearly operate in interaction with environmental factors such as the clinic, the clinician, and the legal and social climate regarding sexuality. Individual practitioners can do little more than to be aware of the factors operating, and seek to actively mitigate them through their interaction with patients, particularly emphasizing genuineness and empathy as well as specifically dealing with their therapeutic acceptance of what patients may consider shameful or abnormal practices.

The imposition of shame and guilt upon sexual interactions by religious and other traditional moralities is the single most important cause of psychological problems in STD treatment, and if the practitioner is able to assess and deal with this early in the treatment process, many difficulties may be prevented or minimized. Lack of consideration may even introduce or reinforce shame or guilt and produce an iatrogenically strengthened psychopathology. A high index of suspicion for psychosocial problems attendant on STD infection or reported infection is mandatory to ensure maximal compliance with treatment, contact tracing or partner notification, prevention and preventive education—and the possible contribution of psychosocial factors to relapse or reinfection should not be underestimated. It can, however, be to some extent neutralized by careful, sympathetic and tactful handling.

In conclusion, it can be demonstrated that psychological aspects of STDs play a central part in understanding the incidence, presentation, treatment and prevention of these diseases. This is particularly true where the infection is not curable or is associated with stigmatization (e.g., genital herpes or HIV infection). In sexual counselling within the context of managing STDS, the psychological aspects of the problem may cause as much or more morbidity and distress as the physical ones, and these reactions need to be understood and treated by the practitioner. Understanding some of the stages and ramifications of STDs (including HIV infection) that are described in this chapter, as well as some of the counselling approaches to them, should place the practitioner in a good position to deal with them in clinical practice. The goals of counselling should include promoting the sexual health of persons with STDs.

REFERENCES

1. Harris, R.D. and Ramsay, A.T. *Health care counselling*. Sydney: Williams & Wilkins, 1988.
2. Hicks, D. A brief history of STDs. *British Journal of Sexual Medicine*, 1994; 21: 32–33.
3. Woolley, P. Psychological responses to a diagnosis of STD. *British Journal of Sexual Medicine*, 1997; 24: 6–8.

4. Cass, V.C. Homosexual identity formation: a theoretical model. *Journal of Homosexuality*, 1979; 4: 19–235.
5. Ross, M.W. Psychosocial factors in admitting to homosexuality in sexually transmitted disease clinics. *Journal of Sexually Transmitted Diseases*, 1985; 12: 83–86.
6. Rosser, B.R.S., Bockting, W.O., Short, B.J. and Ross, M.W. Internalized homophobia and unsafe sex in men who have sex with men. *Abstracts of the 12th World AIDS Conference, Geneva, Switzerland*, 1988, June 28–July 3.
7. Ross, M.W. AIDS phobias: a report of four cases. *Psychopathology*, 1988; 21: 26–30.
8. Salt, H., Miller, R., Perry, L. and Bor, R. Paradoxical interventions in counselling for people with intractable AIDS-worry. *Journal of AIDS Care*, 1989; 1: 38–44.
9. Humphreys, R.A.L. *Tearoom trade: a study of impersonal sex in public places.* London: Duckworth, 1970.
10. Ross, M.W. *The married homosexual man: a psychological study.* London: Routledge & Kegan Paul, 1983.
11. Coleman, E. Developmental stages of the coming-out process. *American Behavioral Scientist*, 1982; 25: 469–482.
12. Drob, S., Leemet, L. and Lifshutz, H. Genital herpes: the psychological consequences. *British Journal of Medical Psychology*, 1985; 58: 307–315.
13. Goldmeir, D. Psychosexual problems. *British Medical Journal*, 1984; 288: 704–705.
14. Aral, S.O., Gates, W. and Jenkins, W.C. Genital herpes: does knowledge lead to action? *American Journal of Public Health*, 1985: 69–71, 75.
15. Rosser, B.R.S. and Ross, M.W. Emotional and life change impact of AIDS on homosexual men in two countries. *Psychology and Health*, 1988; 2: 301–317.
16. Kübler-Ross, E. *On death and dying.* London: Tavistock, 1969.
17. Ross, M.W., Tebble, W.E.M. and Viliunas, D. Staging of reactions to AIDS virus infection in asymptomatic homosexual men. *Journal of Psychology and Human Sexuality*, 1989; 2: 93–104.
18. Rosser, B.R.S., Gobby, J.M. and Carr, W.P. The unsafe sexual behavior of persons living with HIV: An empirical approach to developing new HIV prevention interventions targeting HIV-positive persons. *Journal of Sex Education and Therapy*, 1999, in press.
19. Hart, G. *Sexual maladjustment and disease: an introduction to modern venereology.* Chicago: Nelson-Hall, 1977.
20. Ross, M.W. Illness behavior among patients attending a sexually transmitted disease clinic. *Journal of Sexually Transmitted Diseases*, 1987; 14: 174–179.
21. Catalan J., Bradley, M., Gallwey, J. and Hawton, K. Sexual dysfunction and psychiatric morbidity in patients attending a clinic for sexually transmitted diseases. *British Journal of Psychiatry*, 1981; 138: 292–296.

8 *Sexuality and preventive health care*

In modern medicine, the role of preventive health care is becoming increasingly important as individuals and communities express interest in maintaining some control over their health. The increase in knowledge about the antecedents of disease has also played a part in making preventive education possible, as has the increasing specialization in health and the consequent emphasis on general practitioners and community health centres as being involved in the primary or secondary prevention of disease.

The major areas of sexuality in which prevention of difficulties may occur include contraception, Papanicolaou (Pap) smears and breast self-examination. Other areas that should also be considered are the relationship of drugs to sexuality, sexual education of patients, testicular self-examination, regular prostate examinations for older men, and the dangers of some sex 'toys'. Of these areas, traditionally contraception and family planning is the one most commonly dealt with by practitioners.

CONTRACEPTION

Health services have routinely advised on and prescribed contraception, particularly to women, and the practise of this area of preventive sexual health is not usually controversial in the health care setting. As this has been extensively reviewed elsewhere[1] it will be covered only briefly here.

There is no ideal method of contraception: each method has advantages and disadvantages, and contraception should be tailored to the case of the individual patient. Diamond[1] suggests that the role of the health practitioner is to make clear the relative advantages and disadvantages of each method in the light of the individual's age, health, and medical picture, as well as his or her social situation with regard to a partner, coital frequency and context, maturity, reliability (of both method and patient) and other relevant factors. Usually, contraception is a matter that is the concern of the woman, and in taking any health history the history of contraception will be included. It is a matter that should be raised in every case, and contraception should be reviewed from time to time to determine whether the method used is still the most appropriate if circumstances or medical knowledge change. Contraception is also a useful stepping-off point for raising other areas of sexual preventive health.

SEXUALLY TRANSMISSIBLE DISEASE PREVENTION

The traditional way of preventing STDs has been use of the condom.[2] This is still the case. If male patients are sexually active with more than one partner, then condom use should be advised. While instructions are included with most condoms, the practitioner should assist the patient by discussing the major issues involved with the patient. These include using only water-based lubricant, as oil-based ones will perish the condom; expelling any air remaining in the teat of the condom when putting it on; ensuring that the condom covers the entire shaft of the penis but not the scrotum; and holding the condom in place during withdrawal. Because the adoption of safer-sex practices has been shown to be greater where condoms have been provided at the site of counselling, practitioners may wish to consider offering condoms as part of STD counselling and education. This may do more to decrease the risk of STDs than any other single act the practitioner may perform.

One of the greatest difficulties in advising condom use is the negative attitudes held towards them by some people. Such negative attitudes include the view that it is 'like taking a shower in a raincoat' and the belief that condoms interrupt sexual pleasure and the sexual act. Many of these beliefs are based on the performance of the thicker rubber condoms of past decades (and are often voiced by people who have never used a condom). However, such apparent drawbacks as lessened sensitivity and interruption of sex may also be advantages. Lessened sensation may make the sexual act last longer. Integrating the placement of the condom into foreplay has also been reported as being extremely erotic. Generally, attitudes towards condoms are the greatest barrier to their use, and the practitioner should be prepared to offer information that may change attitudes as well as encouraging the use of condoms or providing a condom for experimentation.

The 'female' condom is still a relatively new advance in technology, which has significant advantages and disadvantages over the 'male' condom. Advantages include the fact that the condom can be inserted prior to sexual activity; enables the receptive partner to directly protect themselves; does not require maintenance of an erection to use; and for men who report decreased sensitivity in using the male condom, provides friction and sensation similar to unprotected sex. Disadvantages include the fact that it is usually more expensive, less familiar to many people, can be a little more difficult to apply, and in some circumstances has been known to produce a squeaking sound during sex. Particularly for women, for men who prefer the receptive position in anal sex, and for men who report difficulties in using male condoms, education about the option of using the 'female' condom as STD prevention can be highly successful in promoting STD prevention.

PREVENTION OR EARLY DETECTION OF CANCER

The Pap smear has been commonly used to detect cervical intra-epithelial neoplasia (CIN) which may develop, if untreated, into carcinoma in situ or disseminated carcinoma. The great majority (90%)[3] of cervical or vulvar higher grades of neoplasia involve subtypes of human papilloma virus (HPV, the genital wart virus); this emphasizes the need both for STD precautions as well as regular Pap smears. Almost all cases of CIN or carcinoma in situ can be successfully treated if detected early. Paavonen and colleagues[3] note that herpes simplex virus (HSV) has also been isolated from tumours of the lower genital tract, although the interactions between HPV and HSV are not fully understood.

From the perspective of preventive health, patients should be told of the relationship between sexually transmissible viruses and cancer of the lower genital tract. What should be emphasized is that by regular Pap smears almost all precancerous abnormalities can be detected and successfully treated (usually on an outpatient basis). Unfortunately, many women are aware of the need for a regular Pap smear but have no idea why they should have one. Simple and straightforward explanation of why people should take particular preventive precautions invariably increases the compliance rate considerably.

Genital warts may also be associated with cancers of other genital sites, most notably the anus and penis. While the risk of progression is significantly greater if there is immunosuppression, people who have had anal warts treated and men with a history of penile warts should be advised to reattend if there appears to be any recurrence. This is particularly important for persons living with HIV. It is debatable whether explicit information on the possibility of malignancies should be provided given their low probability and the desire not to unduly scare people, but certainly the patient should be advised to have a high index of suspicion for regrowth and to attend if further abnormal growths are detected.

Pelvic inflammatory disease (PID) is usually caused by the migration of organisms from the vagina or cervix to the endometrium, fallopian tubes and (or) contiguous structures. It is a major cause of infertility as well as of acute or chronic abdominal pain. Weström and MÅrdh[4] note that most cases of PID are caused by exogenous pathogens such as gonorrhea or chlamydia. The linking of STDs with PID is not well understood by many women, and preventive education must be based on an understanding of what must be prevented and the possible health consequences of infection. Again, this is an area of health promotion that can be simply explained but very frequently is not. We cannot expect patients to take reasonable precautions until the reasons have been explained to them so that they may make an informed decision based on their own motivation rather than on advice.

Most public STD clinics and health departments have a wide range of simple and easy-to-read material on STDs and their signs, consequences and avoidance or treatment, and if the practitioner is serious about preventive health services, these might be obtained either for display in the waiting room or for distribution to patients.

PREVENTION EXAMINATIONS FOR CANCERS

Women

The best known example of self-examination for cancer is breast self-examination. However, it sometimes causes concern because women are unsure what to look for or what it might feel like, and because the subject of cancer is too frightening. Nevertheless, early detection of breast cancer will lead to an increased chance of successful treatment. Women who are at risk of breast cancer by reason of family history, not having had a pregnancy or having their first pregnancy later in life should be advised to regularly examine their breasts. While most lumps detected by breast self-examination prove to be benign, the advantages of early detection of those that prove to be malignant outweigh the disadvantages. Given that around one in ten women will have breast cancer, breast self-examination should be advised and explained to every female patient.

Where it is available, mammography is another service that will detect breast lumps at a size at which they are usually not detectable by self-examination, and this alternative should also be discussed with the patient where appropriate. Ultrasound examinations should also be used in women at high risk.

Men

Testicular cancer is the primary cause of cancer death in men between the ages of 15 and 34. However, it is also one of the most responsive to early treatment, with a success rate exceeding 90% for those without secondary spread.[5] Further, testicular self-examination is easily performed and any abnormalities are usually quite easily detected. Testicular self-examination is thus even more appropriate to advise as a preventive measure than is breast self-examination for women. For some reason, however, it has been virtually ignored by health practitioners and by preventive health services. With male patients who are between adolescence and middle age, testicular self-examination should be advised and the reasons given. Where patients are at higher risk, for example having a history of an undescended testicle, such advice should be mandatory.

While prostate cancer remains a leading cause of death for older men, many men are reluctant to submit to prostate checks, principally from fear of the rectal digital examination. Explaining the need for annual examinations for middle-aged men and older—the precise age recommendations differ between countries—is thus an important part of health care. During a prostate examination, it is usually helpful to explain to the patient what you are doing and why. Simple practice techniques—for example, if the man tenses up, to wait before proceeding and asking the patient to relax—are more helpful than forcing your finger into the rectum. Normalizing reluctance, and specifically discussing common fears (including pain and involuntary sexual response) can also be helpful.

SEX TOYS

This category covers any object that can be inserted into the vagina, anus or urethra. While it is probably an uncommon practice, if patients present with injury suspected to have been caused by insertion of a foreign object into an orifice then advice on the dangers of such practices is appropriate. It seems every emergency room has stories of pens up urethras and bottles or other objects lost in vaginas and/or anuses. While for the novice this can be titillating, for most professionals it soon becomes tiresome and even aggravating. Unfortunately, because the injury is sexually related and many practitioners do not understand the underlying dynamics, some health practitioners can become angry at the patient and even shame the patient—

something they wouldn't think of doing for other repeated problems, such as asthma and broken legs.

How can the health practitioner best help the patient? First, it is important to realize that if the behavior is pleasurable to the patient it will probably continue. Hence, providing *limited information* to the patient on how to lessen harm is appropriate. Objects should be unbreakable, without protrusions which cause trauma, and suitably lubricated. They should also have attachments that allow them to be retrieved. If patients do wish to continue the use of sex toys as part of their erotic repertoire, they should be encouraged to ensure that these toys are appropriate and safe. Using Annon's model, five minutes of mutual discussion on how to pleasure oneself safely is better than a physician-initiated lecture on the subject.

Second, where the person indicates a history of object insertion leading to injury or emergency room visits, the practitioner should suspect that the behavior is compulsive (see chapter 6 on compulsive sexual behavior). This is particularly likely where the patient also reports the behavior as out of voluntary control or finds the behavior distressing. Referral of the person for appropriate assessment and/or treatment with a mental health professional (psychiatrist or psychologist) trained in the treatment of compulsive disorders is indicated. The practitioner should note that the behavior is unlikely to cease without pharmacological and therapy intervention. Hence, the practitioner should not be surprised at the return of patients if the appropriate referral has not been made.

DRUGS AND ALCOHOL

Drugs are frequently used in association with sexual contact, with alcohol probably being the most common. In the younger age group, so-called 'party drugs' (amphetamines and their derivatives) may also be used, and the use of volatile nitrites to enhance orgasm is common, particularly by men when engaging in anal intercourse (insertive or receptive). These drugs may be used simultaneously.

While drugs may have their own negative effects if taken in inappropriate doses, their prime risk with regard to sexual behavior (see also chapter 10 on drugs and sexual functioning) is that of clouding judgment and causing disinhibition.

Where judgment is clouded, risks are taken that would not normally occur. Chief among these risks are having intercourse when it would not normally occur, and having intercourse without protection (either contraception or more probably protection from STDs). When a sexual history is taken, co-factors such as drugs should be ascertained; if drug use appears to be related to risk behaviors, then the practitioner should note this. The patient may have no conscious awareness of the part drug use may play in initiating sexual contact, or of its relationship with particularly risky behaviors. If this appears to be the case, then the practitioner should advise the patient of the risks involved where judgment is clouded. Unfortunately, alcohol and other drugs may be so closely associated with sexual contacts— both because of their disinhibiting action and because of the traditional relationship between sex and celebrations or bars and dances as places for making sexual contact—that awareness may not be translated into action.

It can be seen from these examples that there is considerable scope for the practitioner to engage in preventive health measures with patients in the area of sexual functioning. Generally raising the issue of preventive health care may also be a useful way of moving into the area of taking a sexual history. Of course, where an STD has been diagnosed, preventive education is mandatory (as described in chapter 11, which discusses pre- and post-test counselling). However, preventive education in the area of sexual health should be seen as a part of general preventive health and medicine, and integrated into general patient and community primary prevention of health problems. In this context, a simple explanation of what can be prevented and why is a useful stimulus to motivating the patient to look after his or her own health, and to promoting attendance for regular screening as appropriate.

REFERENCES

1. Diamond, M. Sex and reproduction: conception and contraception. In Green, R. (ed.) *Human sexuality: a health practitioner's text.* (2nd edn). Baltimore: Williams & Wilkins, 1979: 58–80.
2. Brandt, A.M. *No magic bullet: a social history of venereal diseases in the United States since 1880.* New York: Oxford University Press, 1985.
3. Paavonen, J., Koutsky, L.A. and Kiviat, N. Cervical neoplasms and other STD-related genital and anal neoplasms. In Holmes, K.K., MÅrdh, P.A., Sparling, P.F. and Wiesner, P.J. (eds) *Sexually transmitted diseases.* (2nd edn). New York: McGraw-Hill, 1990: 561–592.
4. Weström, L. and MÅrdh, P.A. Acute pelvic inflammatory disease. In Holmes, K.K, MÅrdh, P.A., Sparling, P.F. and Wiesner, P.J. (eds) *Sexually transmitted diseases.* (2nd edn). New York: McGraw-Hill, 1990: 593–613.
5. Anderson, E.E. Early diagnosis of testicular carcinoma: self-examination of the testicle. *North Carolina Medical Journal,* 1985; 46: 407–409.

9 *Sexuality and chronic illness*

Although many chronic illnesses have an effect on sexuality, patients are notoriously reluctant to discuss the issue unless it is broached by a practitioner. Studies of patient populations show that while many patients report sexual problems when specifically asked about them, few have mentioned them to their health practitioner.[1] This may be a matter of reticence, or a preoccupation with more pressing concerns such as the possibility of a terminal illness.

It is therefore incumbent on practitioners to introduce the question of the effect of illness on the patient's sexuality. Perhaps the best way to introduce the subject is to use a 'normalizing' approach such as, 'Many people with your illness find they have some sexual problems. Have you noticed any difficulties since your illness began?'.

Responses to this kind of advance vary enormously. A cheery couple in late middle age nodded happily to each other as the husband said, 'Oh, we're past all that, love'. A young married man who had had consultations with a broad range of health practitioners before reaching the pain clinic of a large public hospital was moved almost to tears. 'That's the very worst thing going wrong in my life and no one's ever asked me about it before.' We have also been told to mind our own business.

The implication is plain. The issue needs to be broached in all cases of chronic illness, but health practitioners need to be sensitive to the fact that some patients will not have a problem and some will be simply unwilling to discuss any difficulties. The patient must, however, be given the choice.

Chronic illness can have both physical and psychological effects on sexuality. Box 9-1 lists some illnesses that frequently have physical effects on sexual performance and enjoyment.

PSYCHIATRIC DISORDERS AND SEXUALITY

Analysis of the impact of psychiatric disorder on sexuality is difficult because of the confounding effects of medication. It is often hard to assess whether sexual dysfunction is a direct result of the psychiatric disorder or a side effect of the long-term use of psychotropic drugs.

BOX 9-1
Chronic illness and sex

Arthritis	Pain may make intercourse difficult. Involvement of the hip particularly may preclude intercourse.[5]
Asthma	Sexual arousal may be associated with attacks. A feedback loop may be set up with the patient becoming anxious and increasing the chances of an attack.[6]
Chronic benign pain	Reduction in intercourse frequency because of pain.[7]
Diabetes	While libido usually remains intact, about 50% of diabetic men suffer a degree of erectile dysfunction.[8]
Multiple sclerosis	Demyelination of neurones can affect erectile capacity, ejaculation, orgasm and movement.
Neurological damage	Many effects, depending on site, size and side of lesion.
Obstructive airways disease	Breathlessness detracts from sexual performance and enjoyment.[9]
Renal disease	Patients report loss of libido, anorgasmia and erectile dysfunction.[10]
Sleep apnea	40% of male patients report erectile dysfunction. Moodiness disrupts relationships.[11]
Spinal injury	Depending on the level of injury, some or all of sexual sensation and function may belost in both sexes.
Vascular disease	About half of male patients suffering from reduced blood circulation in the legs show erectile dysfunction.[12] Antihypertensive drugs may also cause dysfunction.[13]

Loss of libido is one of the classic symptoms of severe depression. This will have an impact on sexual relationships. It is worth remembering that depression features in many cases of chronic illness and that both monoamine oxidase inhibitors and tricyclic antidepressants have been found to reduce erectile and ejaculatory capacity.[2]

Some schizophrenic patients focus their delusions and hallucinations on sexual matters. More commonly, there is a reduction in sexual interest and fantasy. Nestoros, Lehmann and Ban[3] studied hospitalized, medicated, schizophrenic patients and found that many reported having no interest whatsoever in sexuality. A further confounding factor here is that many schizophrenic patients are socially withdrawn and hence unlikely to find a partner. Also, the policy of most psychiatric hospitals has been to discourage sexual activity between patients.

Substance abuse is usually deleterious to sexual well-being. Both acute and chronic alcohol overuse reduce the male's capacity for penile erection and the female's orgasmic capacity.

Barbiturates and stimulants can both affect sexual performance negatively. There have been some claims for an aphrodisiac effect from LSD, but the effect of the drug is unreliable. Similarly some people find that marijuana enhances sexual pleasure, specifically of orgasm.

PSYCHOSOCIAL EFFECTS OF CHRONIC ILLNESS

Changes in appearance either as a result of the illness or of treatment can be devastating to a person's sexual self-image. Hair loss resulting from chemotherapy, the surgical removal of a body part and so on can have a major impact. The patient feels unattractive and may assume that the partner will not welcome sexual advances.

Many chronically ill patients feel lethargic and simply cannot summon up the energy for intercourse. Especially for patients recovering from stroke or myocardial infarct, there may be a fear that sexual activity will increase the risk of a second attack. The patient needs to be reassured that sexual activity, like any other form of moderate exercise, is actually beneficial to the cardiovascular system.

There is a need for careful inquiry about the effect of illness on the patient's relationship, as people vary tremendously in their response to illness. It may very well be a good idea to talk to the couple together (see chapter 5) as the partners may not have communicated frankly and may have quite erroneous impressions of what the other person is thinking and feeling.

For the patient who has a visible disability, but no partner, the effects on sexuality may be intensified. Gill[14] describes the problems of spinal cord injured women in attracting partners as a 'romantic disadvantage'. She notes that such women who have once had difficulties in a relationship with a 'normal' partner may tend to be drawn to partners in a minority group, such as other disabled persons or members of socially-disadvantaged ethnic groups.

Box 9-2 gives some common responses of patients and partners.

SEXUAL REHABILITATION

Dengrove[4] outlines some important factors in rehabilitation. First, the quality of the sexual relationship before the illness is important. If the relationship had been a good one, one or both partners may feel deprived by the loss of a fulfilling part of life. If the relationship had been poor, one or both may use the illness as an excuse for ceasing the sexual relationship altogether.

Secondly, the physical effects of the illness influence the extent to which rehabilitation is possible. As outlined in Box 9-1, many illnesses have direct effects on sexuality and libido. Others produce tiredness and a general lack of motivation, which includes sexual motivation.

Thirdly, the person's response to the illness in terms of its impact on sexual self-image is relevant. A woman who has had a radical mastectomy may feel very much less of a sexual being after the operation.

Various therapies may affect sexual function and sexual image. Medication may reduce erectile ability, reduce orgasmic capacity or lessen libido. Surgery such as mastectomy and hysterectomy may affect sexual self-image in women. Chemotherapy with its associated hair loss may make the patient feel unattractive or make the partner perceive the patient as sexually unattractive. It also tends to produce lethargy, which reduces the likelihood of the patient's engaging in sexual activity.

Lastly, the response of the patient and partner as a couple is relevant (see Box 9-2).

Ducharme and Gill's[15] useful handbook on sexual rehabilitation after spinal cord injury has a broader relevance to other situations. Its question and answer format is primarily aimed at patients, but it is informative for professionals too.

These factors all need to be assessed, preferably with the patient and partner together. The couple may need the first three steps of the PLISSIT model—permission to discuss the issues, limited information and specific suggestions.

BOX 9-2
Partnership responses to chronic illness

Responses from the patient

1. Concern about how the partner will feel about reduced sexual activity.
2. Anger, repressed or felt, that the partner is still healthy.
3. Guilt. The illness is a punishment and the patient deserves to lose the pleasures of sexuality.
4. Sexual frustration. This is especially so in a sexually functioning patient who requires long periods of hospitalization. Most hospitals pay little if any attention to the sexual needs of patients.
5. Use of the illness to break off sexual relations completely if the relationship was previously unsatisfactory.
6. Worries about possible infidelity by a frustrated partner.
7. Anxiety about possible sexual failure.
8. Concerns that changes in appearance may be unattractive.

Responses from the partner

1. Sexual frustration. This may lead to searching for another partner.
2. Anger because of deprivation.
3. Resentment of increased service demands.
4. Worry that sexual activity may damage the patient's health.
5. Use of the illness to break off sexual relations where they have previously been less than satisfactory.
6. Guilt that he or she, the partner, is not sick.
7. Distaste about changes in the patient's appearance.
8. An irrational belief that sexual relations may be a means of contagion, especially seen when the patient has cancer.

Specialized facilities may be available, such a those for 'sexual rediscovery' in women with spinal cord injury[16]. It is the responsibility of the professional to seek out any programs available in their local area as the need arises. A client who feels you are not giving up on them, even if you personally do not have expertise in the area, will be more optimistic and hopeful of a positive outcome.

REFERENCES

1. Schover, L.R. and Jensen, S.B. *Sexuality and chronic illness. A comprehensive approach.* New York: The Guilford Press, 1988.

2. Dickes, R. and Fleming, J.L. Sexuality in general medical practice. In Simons, R.C. (ed.) *Understanding human behaviour in health and illness.* (3rd edn). Baltimore: Williams & Wilkins, 1985.

3. Nestoros, J.N., Lehmann, H.E. and Ban, T.A. Sexual behaviour of the male schizophrenic: The impact of illness and medications. *Archives of Sexual Behaviour*, 1981; 10: 421–442.

4. Dengrove, E. Sexual responses to disease processes. *Journal of Sex Research*, 1968; 4: 257–264.

5. Ehrlich, G.E. Sexual problems and the arthritic patient. In Ehrlich, G.E. (ed.) *Total management of the arthritic patient.* Philadelphia: J.B. Lippincott, 1973.

6. Kaplan, R.M., Reis, A. and Atkins, C.J. Behavioural issues in the management of chronic obstructive pulmonary disease. *Annals of Behavioural Medicine*, 1985; 7: 5–10.

7. Sjogren, K. and Fugl-Meyer, A.R. Chronic back pain and sexuality. *Journal of Rehabilitation Medicine*, 1981; 3: 19–25.

8. Ellenberg, M. Impotence and diabetes mellitus: the neurological factor. *Annals of Internal Medicine*, 1971; 75: 213–219.

9. Hanson, E.I. Effects of chronic lung disease on life in general and on sexuality: perceptions of adult patients. *Heart and Lung*, 1982; 11: 435–431.

10. Abram, H.S. Sexual functioning in patients with chronic renal failure. *Journal of Nervous and Mental Disease*, 1975; 160: 220–226.

11. Singh, B. Sleep apnea: A psychiatric perspective. In Saunders, N.A. and Sullivan, C.E. (eds) *Sleep and breathing.* New York: Marcel Dekker, Inc., 1984.

12. Metz, P. Erectile dysfunction in men with occlusive arterial disease in the legs. *Danish Medical Bulletin*, 1983; 30: 185–189.

13. Moss, H.B. and Procci, W.R. Sexual dysfunction associated with oral antihypertensive medication: A critical survey of the literature. *General Hospital Psychiatry*, 1982; 4: 121–129.

14. Gill, C. Dating and relationships. In Krotoski, D.M., Nosek, M.A. and Turk, M.A. *Women with physical disabilities: Achieving and maintaining health and well-being.* Baltimore: Paul H. Brookes, 1996.

15. Ducharme, S.H. and Gill, K.M. *Sexuality after spinal cord injury: Answers to your questions.* Baltimore: Paul H. Brookes, 1997.

16. Whipple, B., Richards, E. and others. Sexual response in women with complete spinal cord injury. In Krotski, D.M., Nosek, M.A. and Turk, M.A. *Women with physical disabilities: Achieving and maintaining health and well-being.* Baltimore: Paul H. Brookes, 1996.

10 *Sexuality and drug-related history*

A number of drugs, both prescribed and social, may have an effect on sexual functioning. Such effects may be due to the direct action of the drug or to an interaction between the drug and psychological factors; or, in the case of prescribed drugs, the effects may be a response to the illness for which the drug has been prescribed rather than being caused by the drug itself.

It is not commonly appreciated that there may be an iatrogenic component to sexual dysfunctions. This may be through direct and indirect effects (e.g., through its effects on libido, rather than on the physiology of sexual function) and appears more likely to affect male function than female function. The possibility of iatrogenic factors influencing or causing sexual dysfunction, as well as the fact that social drugs may also have the same effects, should make a history of medication and drug use mandatory when you are investigating sexual dysfunction. There are a number of ways drugs may affect sexual function.

CENTRAL NERVOUS SYSTEM (CNS) DEPRESSANTS

Alcohol is the best known and probably most commonly implicated example of a CNS depressant with potential effects on sexual function. CNS depressants may act by reducing libido and causing sexual dysfunction secondary to this. However, the effect may be variable; for example, a small amount of alcohol may increase libido but larger amounts decrease it. Alcohol in larger quantities has the classic acute effect of increasing desire but decreasing performance. Chronic alcohol use may not affect libido to the same extent as acute intoxication but is often associated with impotence. Chronic alcohol abuse may cause liver dysfunction—which can then affect hormonal function, leading in extreme cases to feminization in men—or, through damage to the peripheral nervous system, may interfere with the physical component of erection. Disturbance of the pituitary-gonadal axis from chronic alcohol consumption may also impair sexual response.

While CNS depressants may attenuate libido—and there is some suggestion that oral contraceptives in women may also reduce libido—in small doses anxiolytics may, like alcohol, initially increase libido but in larger doses reduce it.

OTHER DRUGS

Opioids: Opioids may have a complex effect on sexual function. In addition to their effect on CNS function, they will have a sedative effect and will increase prolactin release, which will in turn inhibit sexual function.

Antihypertensives: Some antihypertensives (e.g., thiazide diuretics) have been implicated in erectile dysfunction and may also interfere with ejaculation (adrenergic neuron blockers). Some, such as methyldopa and clonidine, have their influence by acting as CNS *depressants.* Beta blockers have only minor effects on sexual function. Drugs that interfere with the sympathetic nervous system may cause failure of ejaculation and secondarily, via psychological mechanisms, sexual dysfunction.

Anticholinergic agents: Many drugs have anticholinergic properties, and thus may have an effect on sexual function by interfering with erection, which is dependent on sacral parasympathetic function. Tricyclic antidepressants and some of the classical antipsychotic agents such as chlorpromazine and thioridazine may have this effect. Classical antihistamine agents such as antimotion sickness preparations may also affect sexual function in the same way, as well as through their sedating effects.

Agents that increase prolactin secretion: Such agents decrease the release of gonadotrophins from the pituitary and thus, secondarily, decrease gonadal hormone release. This ultimately is associated with decreased libido and secondary sexual dysfunction. The commonest mechanism for increasing prolactin is by blockade of dopamine receptors in the hypothalamus by drugs such as antipsychotics and also the antiemetic metoclopramide.

There are a number of other drugs that have been associated with sexual dysfunction, although the mechanisms for their effect are not necessarily understood. There is some suggestion from large controlled trials of the treatment of hypertension that thiazide diuretics may increase the incidence of erectile dysfunction, and that overdose of levodopa in Parkinsonian men has resulted in sexual disinhibition—this suggests that dopamine is involved as a neurotransmitter in mediating sexual response. Other drugs that have been reported to affect sexual functioning include some antimigraine preparations, and H2 blockers such as cimetidine.

HORMONES

In the male, anti-androgens will decrease sexual functioning. They operate by reducing libido and thus causing secondary erectile dysfunction. Such drugs (progesterone analogues) may be given to sexual offenders to reduce libido. In general, any agent that decreases testicular function (and thus the production of testosterone), such as cytotoxic agents for treatment of malignancies, will have an effect on sexual function. Provision of androgens to normal males will have no physical effect, although in androgen-deficient men androgen supplementation will increase libido. Similarly, oestrogens in normal women will have no effect on sexual functioning, although in post-menopausal women they may increase vaginal lubrication and thus have a secondary effect on sexual function by making intercourse less painful.

SOCIAL DRUGS

Sexual function may be affected by social drugs, the most common of which is alcohol. However, illicit opioid users will also experience the effects noted above for opioids. The more widespread use of illicit amphetamines also deserves consideration. There have been reports that there is a heightening of sexual interest when coming down from some amphetamines (particularly methamphetamines), and other amphetamine users have reported these drugs enhance sexual experience. However, there has been little systematic work on this class of agents from the sexual direction.

The literature on cannabis provides conflicting data on many aspects of its use. However, one study does suggest that there may be a higher incidence of erectile dysfunction and decrease in sperm production. Volatile nitrites, inhaled by some homosexual men to heighten the experience of orgasm, do not appear to alter sexual function.

The role of social drugs should be considered not only in relation to their direct effects on sexual function but also in relation to their indirect effects in accompanying sexual behavior, which may be unsafe (in terms of STD and HIV transmission), and in disinhibiting individuals who may have sexual relationships or engage in sexual acts they may otherwise not take part in. Thus, any STD history should also be accompanied by a history of the pharmacological climate of the risk behaviors.

CLINICAL CONSIDERATIONS

Clinically, a proportion of presentations of sexual dysfunction will be psychogenic. Such patients will include people who are on medication that has no direct effect on their sexual functioning. However, it is important for the practitioner to exclude pharmacological factors which may either primarily or secondarily affect sexual functioning, and to consider both prescribed and socially used agents. Drugs may affect different aspects of sexual functioning, and the health practitioner should be aware of the different ways in which particular agents may impact on sexual response. There may also be a spurious association of drugs and sexual functioning secondary to the illness being treated (see particularly the previous chapter on the effect of chronic illness on sexuality) rather than a cause and effect relationship. In relation to general treatment, it should also be noted that if an agent does affect sexual functioning, then this will often affect compliance with the drug regimen.

In conclusion, health practitioners should maintain a high index of suspicion for possible iatrogenic contributions to sexual dysfunction and this index of suspicion should extend to socially used drugs. It is important to exclude pharmacological and physical factors when considering the differential diagnoses for sexual dysfunctions, and this should include taking a drug-use history during the sexual history.

11   *Pre-test and post-test HIV counselling*

The issue of appropriate pre- and post-test screening and counselling has a number of implications for correct counselling and management. For major problems such as HIV (and to a lesser extent, genital herpes) which at present can be controlled but not cured, adequate preparation serves both a preventive role in educating the patient to avoid further transmitting the infection, and prepares for and mitigates the major psychosocial morbidity that may arise from receiving a positive result. In some areas, adequate pre- and post-test counselling for HIV is mandatory by law. Thus for reasons of both law and good practice as well as preventive health care, pre- and post-test counselling is an important part of clinical practice for the management of viral STDs.

PRE-TEST COUNSELLING FOR HIV SCREENING

Screening for antibodies to the human immunodeficiency virus (HIV) has become a reasonably common procedure since the test became available in April 1985. The more recent awareness that knowledge of HIV antibody status (or knowledge of status as a person with herpes) may be detrimental to an individual's mental health has, however, developed more slowly, although it is now well recognized (Goldmeier and colleagues, 1988 for herpes; Ross and Rosser, 1988 for HIV infection).[1,2] In about one third of cases the general practitioner is the point of testing, but little attention has been given to the practicalities of pre-test counselling or the medical and ethical considerations attendant on testing. Box 11-1 provides sample questions to ask when discussing HIV risk with patients.

Screening versus diagnostic testing

A distinction must be made between diagnostic testing and screening, since the ethical considerations are somewhat different. Further, diagnostic testing will be applicable to HIV and herpes, while screening is applicable

BOX 11-1
HIV/STD risk assessment

A. General screen
- Have you had a blood transfusion before 1985?
- Are you a haemophiliac?
- Have you used injecting drugs even once in your life?
- Have you had sex with a partner who you think can answer 'yes' to any of these questions?

B. Sexual risk screen
Do you engage in sex activities involving:
- Anal penetration? (Probes: Giving, receiving, or both? About how often do you use condoms for anal sex, giving or receiving/receptive or insertive?)
- Vaginal penetration? (Probes: About how often do you use condoms for vaginal sex?)
- Oral-genital contact? (Probes: For fellatio, ask: sucking, being sucked or both? About how often do you use condoms for oral sex? For cunnilingus, ask: eating out, being eaten out or both? About how often do you use a barrier, e.g. a dental dam, to protect you when eating out/being eaten out?)
- Oral-anal contact, sometimes called 'rimming'. (Probes: Do you prefer rimming, being rimmed or both? About how often do you use a barrier, e.g. a dental dam, when rimming?)

C. Prevention behavioral screen
- How do you normally protect yourself from getting infected / infecting others with HIV?
- Are there any risk situations that have happened that may be concerning you? (If yes, probe: Tell me what happened.)
- Why do you think you may be infected with HIV?
- Have you had an HIV test before? (Probe: How many times?)
- What would help you to lower your risk in the future?
- Whether this test comes back positive or negative, how are you going to protect yourself in sex in the future?
- Do you need any condoms (needles) or is there anything else I can do to assist you to practise safer sex?

—continued overleaf

BOX 11-1— *continued*

D. Predictive questions

- Do you think your test is going to come back HIV positive or HIV negative? (Probe: Why?)
- How do you think you would handle it if the test did come back positive? (Probe: How have you handled other challenges in your life, e.g., 'coming out'?)

to HIV. Screening describes the process of testing to provide early detection and treatment of a condition. In the case of HIV, since the advent of protease inhibitors, clear benefit for most patients from knowing their HIV serostatus exists. However, benefits must be weighed against potential disadvantages. Where the patient's knowledge of his or her seropositive status may lead to adverse psychological sequelae, then the principle *primum non nocere* (above all, do no harm) should apply, and the test be avoided. Hence, HIV testing should never be automatic or routine.

Knowledge of viral STD infection usually leads the individual to modify lifestyle factors to prevent viral transmission. However, there have also been cases reported where the opposite has occurred, and individuals have set out to infect others, either deliberately or unconsciously, in their anger at finding themselves seropositive.[3] The general practitioner must therefore make a decision as to whether HIV antibody screening is indicated for the individual patient in terms of its probable sequelae. Such reactions also make one of the strongest cases for adequate pre- and post-test counselling.

Diagnostic testing is easier to justify than screening because in most cases it conveys an advantage in permitting differential diagnosis (which may include HIV infection, or herpes infection) and treatment of infections to proceed. Nevertheless, even in this circumstance, the practitioner must still be aware of the potential psychosocial consequences, and with the patient must decide what pre-test counselling is appropriate and how the person should be informed of the results. We present here a guide to how HIV counselling (and to a lesser extent herpes counselling) should proceed in health practice, and a discussion of the considerations underlying this model. These are arranged in the suggested order of counselling and under major areas to cover. While we refer to HIV as the exemplar because it is the most extreme situation, the arguments also apply (although usually with a lesser level of stigma and with a non-fatal outcome) for genital herpes simplex infection. Where herpes differs, this is noted. Otherwise, what is described for HIV will also apply—although without quite the same degree of emotional trauma overall—for herpes.

Reasons to test

Most patients will present specifically requesting the HIV test. It is important to ascertain whether testing is necessary, since there has been extensive media coverage both nationally and internationally (most recently for HIV; in the early 1980s for herpes) that has led to many misconceptions and, in some cases, hysteria. Further, some individuals may present in the absence of any risk. There are three other important reasons for ascertaining a need for testing:

1. The practitioner has an obligation in terms of primary prevention to provide information that ensures that patients do not transmit the virus if they are infected (and do not acquire STD viral infection if they are uninfected).
2. If individuals are AIDS or STD phobic,[4] testing may reinforce their irrational disease conviction.
3. Some patients use HIV testing as a substitute for risk behavior modification, and hence testing can serve as an excuse not to change behavior.

The first step is thus to determine whether the test is appropriate and whether patients may have been exposed to infection.

Risk-taking behaviors

It is important not to phrase the query about risks of infection in terms of 'risk groups'. While, epidemiologically, certain groups show a greater prevalence of HIV or herpes infection, the statistical inference from a population to an individual is not valid, and may lead both to advising testing where inappropriate and not testing where it would be appropriate. Some individuals may, for example, be homosexual but at no risk by virtue of their specific sexual practices.[5] Others may consider themselves heterosexual but nevertheless engage in same-sex practices: Kinsey, Pomeroy and Martin[6] found that 37% of men had had at least one homosexual encounter to orgasm between the ages of 16 and 65 years. Still others may be unaware of their partner's lifestyle or past experience, which in turn has placed them at risk.

Patients should initially be asked what specific behaviors or practices have put them at risk of viral infection. These include:

- Having genital sexual intercourse (anal or vaginal) with more than one partner
- Being the partner of someone at risk
- Sharing needles during injecting drug use
- Having a transfusion of blood or blood products up to April 1985, or a transfusion in Africa and India post-1985
- Being subject to a needlestick injury or mucocutaneous exposure to an HIV seropositive (or possibly seropositive) individual
- Practising oral sexual intercourse (considered low risk)
- Being artificially inseminated with semen from an untested donor
- In pediatric cases, the mother being virus seropositive pre- or peri-natally.

While genital or oral sexual intercourse with condoms markedly reduces risk of infection, cases have been reported where condoms did not provide protection against HIV infection.[7] Where condoms are inappropriately used or of inferior quality, the risk of infection may increase by a factor of ten.[8]

Reaction to test

Many individuals request the HIV antibody test on the assumption that they will be seronegative. Often they will not have thought about the possibility of a positive result. It is imperative to ask what their reaction would be if the test proved to be positive. Their response to this question is one of the best indicators of their actual post-seropositive reaction, and serves both to alert patients to the possibility of negative sequelae, and to introduce them to the fact that there may be negative and harmful consequences arising from a screening test. Response to this question should also alert the practitioner both to potential psychological difficulties if the result proves positive, and to factors that may contraindicate the test. Where patients indicate they would cause themselves or others harm, the practitioner should work with them to develop a realistic plan for coping prior to the test being undertaken.

Coping mechanisms

It is important to gain some insight into the patient's previous mechanisms of coping with stress, as this will provide one of the best indicators of how the individual will cope with a positive test result. Answers to the questions, 'What major stresses have you had in your life to date? How did (or would) you cope with them?' alert the practitioner to the potential need for support following a confirmed test result, and to possible psychological decompensation, suicide attempt, refuge in alcohol or other drugs, or denial. If you believe the patient's life may be at risk following advice of a positive result, or that the life of a third party may be at risk, you should again give very serious consideration to not carrying out the test or, if the test is carried out, to providing appropriate support for the patient.

Concurrent stressors affecting the patient should also be investigated. Clinical experience has demonstrated that a positive HIV antibody or herpes test result may exacerbate any current difficulty in functioning. Specifically, major crises in the last 12 months prior to testing should be investigated, and where they are present and unresolved, testing is usually contraindicated.

Social supports

One of the best predictors of longer term mental health is the degree of social support available to the individual. It is important for the practitioner to ascertain what social supports are available to the patient and any possible complications that may arise from the need to confide in inappropriate individuals. Choice of inappropriate support may lead to discrimination and further distress. Examples of this include confiding in individuals who then broadcast the fact that the patient 'has AIDS' or 'has herpes', and consequent discrimination in or eviction from accommodation, or harassment at or dismissal from employment. Confiding in inappropriate individuals may also lead to the partial or complete loss of social supports at the time when the individual is most in need of them, with potentially serious consequences for mental health. The clinician may need to give consideration to providing such support or referral to agencies that provide support.

Mental history

If responses to the questions discussed above (relating to how the patient would cope with a positive test result, coping with previous stresses, and social supports) reveal evidence that the patient may be at risk physically or psychologically from a positive result, then further details should be sought. Such details will include previous history of mental illness, suicidal ideation or suicide attempts, treatment for anxiety or depression, psychotherapy, psychosis and patterns of compulsive sexual behavior. Any history of severe depression with suicidal ideation, or of psychosis, will raise serious questions as to the advisability of screening. If the test is indicated in differential diagnosis and a positive result is found, it is advisable to have adequate psychological follow-up and a high index of suspicion for changes in psychological state.

Provision of education

In the absence of a cure or vaccine for HIV or herpes infection in the immediate future, there is an absolute obligation for the health practitioner to provide education and to enhance the patient's primary preventive techniques. In addition to questions the patient may have raised in the course of the consultation, the following information must be provided as an absolute minimum:

- A positive HIV antibody test or herpes diagnostic test result indicates that the individual has been infected, is currently infected, and is likely to remain infectious for life.
- A person who is HIV antibody positive or herpes positive is infectious to others, but only under certain circumstances where there is transfer of body fluids (particularly blood, semen and vaginal secretions).
- The individual has an obligation not to infect others if infected, and if uninfected should take all possible steps to remain that way. These steps include avoidance of unsafe sex in which transfer of body fluids may occur, and not sharing needles during injecting drug use. Reduction of sexual partners to a minimum and use of condoms to reduce risk of infection should be advised.

This information should be provided before testing, and certainly prior to the provision of the test result. Information provided at the same time as the test result is usually not remembered in the euphoria of a negative result or lost in the shock of a positive result.

Informed consent

The fact that HIV screening may have negative consequences for the individual should be discussed with the patient for consent to be fully informed. The following areas must be covered:

- There is no cure currently available. Available treatments can reduce progression of disease.
- A positive result for many persons reduces risk behaviors, but this is not universal. There is thus advantage to some people, but not necessarily the individual, in taking the test.
- The result of a positive test may lead to psychological decompensation (breakdown or inability to cope), depression and anxiety.
- The person must be made aware of the relevant laws relating to notification and penalties associated with transmission of the virus.
- The patient must be made aware of the potential infringement of rights (loss of housing, employment) arising from potential breaches of

confidentiality, and the potential disadvantages of divulging positive HIV antibody status to third parties.

- Life insurance may not be available to individuals who are HIV antibody positive.

As with other medical procedures, however, consent is not held to be informed if potential disadvantages are not discussed. Although to date there have not been any cases to provide guidelines, there are a number of potential medicolegal issues involved in HIV antibody testing, with informed consent and the basis of the clinical decision to carry out testing being the two most prominent issues.

Preventive counselling

In the absence of a cure, the health practitioner has an obligation to encourage primary prevention in those who present, both those specifically seeking the HIV antibody and/or herpes diagnostic testing and others whose behaviors put them at risk of infection. It must be noted that testing is not essential to prevention, for if all individuals avoided behaviors that put them at risk of HIV infection, the spread of this epidemic would cease.

In our experience, people who present for testing want specific advice to lower their risk. It is insufficient to simply advise them to 'use condoms in the future'. By the time the person presents, she or he already know this information. Central to the prevention of the virus's spread is development of an effective and realistic prevention plan individualized to meet each person's circumstances (see chapter 7). For example, Rosser[9] demonstrated that in response to HIV, gay men tend to adopt one of three distinct strategies: risk avoidance (no anal intercourse); risk substitution (condom use for all penetrative sex); and contextual modification (adoption of sexual monogamy at least for anal intercourse). Asking how the person plans to prevent future risks of infection is helpful. Working with the patient, one can then develop an appropriate plan, if necessary with a back-up plan. For example, the businessman who presents for testing because he had a 'fling' while on a business trip may propose future monogamy to reduce risk. One can affirm such resolutions where realistic, while still recommending he take condoms on future trips 'just in case'. The hallmarks of traditional STD prevention—advocacy of condoms and advice to reduce the number of partners—then can be tailored to individuals' circumstances.

Advice on condom use needs to be specific, behaviorally oriented, and demonstrated where possible (see chapter 7). Research into heterosexual use of condoms shows that when used properly, failure rate is less than 3/100 woman years, although in general usage it may rise to 10/100 woman years.[10]

For injecting drug users, research confirms that ensuring access to needles effectively prevents HIV spread while not increasing drug use. Hence, offering needle access together with help to enter treatment is now the standard in prevention intervention. In areas where needle access is still prohibited, practitioners may provide advice on the necessity of not sharing needles and also information on how to sterilize equipment, although these are less effective than needle access programs.

Where a simple behavioral plan appears unlikely to prevent risk, or where the person appears resistant to developing an effective plan, the practitioner should consider referral; for example, to a qualified mental health professional, HIV prevention case manager, or sex therapist. Patients who say they cannot stop having sex when they go out, or are so depressed they don't care, or are insecure about using condoms, should be seen as needing professional help beyond the skills of most practitioners.

Efficacy of testing on behavioral change

The assumption is frequently made that testing for HIV will encourage individuals to prevent or avoid viral transmission. The evidence on this is ambiguous, with one study showing that while individuals who are seropositive reduce partner numbers by up to 50%, seronegative individuals show little reduction. On the other hand, further studies have showed that individuals who did not know their antibody status after testing showed no reduction in partner numbers. A comparison of the effects of counselling alone, testing alone, testing plus counselling, and no intervention, with regard to AIDS prophylactic behaviors in homosexual men, found that counselling and testing were more effective than testing only, which in turn was more effective than counselling alone, which had more effect than no intervention.[11]

It would seem reasonable to conclude that counselling does enhance the effect of testing, and that testing may have benefits in terms of reduction of viral spread. However, the role of the health practitioner is to identify those individuals for whom testing would be advantageous, and to refer on for a further opinion those for whom a positive test result would lead to harm or to increased viral transmission. For those who may be harmed by a positive test result, but for whom the medical practitioner believes the test to be appropriate, more intensive follow-up and support is recommended.

Other sexually transmitted diseases

If a patient is judged to be at risk of HIV infection through sexual contact or genital herpes infection, then he or she will also be at risk from other sexually transmissible diseases (STDs). It is important for the practitioner to be aware of this and to concurrently test for other diseases. This should include syphilis serology, hepatitis B serology, and urine testing for gonorrhea and chlamydia. If the practitioner does not feel competent to carry out full venereological examination, referral should be made to a local STD clinic. It is important not to forget that HIV is primarily an STD and that, while patients may not be infected with HIV, they may carry other STDs that require treatment. The high proportion of STDs that are asymptomatic reinforces the importance of such concurrent screening.

Recording HIV tests and results

The possibility of discrimination (real or imagined) against patients, if their results were to be disclosed to others, has led to considerable concern about confidentiality. This may include concern about results being communicated to reception staff or to members of the patient's family or to the spouse (particularly where family members are seen by the same practitioner or at the same practice). Reassurance of confidentiality is therefore appropriate. Common practices to ensure confidentiality may include providing a code (or alias) on specimens or request forms, and keeping a private or locked register of such codes or aliases. Recording of results on patient files has not provided adequate protection of confidentiality in some hospital settings[12] and may be similarly inadequate in private settings or where many personnel have access to patient files. These issues do need to be considered and patients may request specific reassurance on matters of confidentiality which we are accustomed to take for granted.

POST-TEST COUNSELLING FOR HIV SCREENING

Post-test counselling is complementary to pre-test counselling, and the counselling described here is that which will follow such pre-test counselling. Again, we use HIV infection as the exemplar but find this to be equally applicable to genital herpes infection (although there is usually less trauma involved). It must be emphasized that results for HIV should not be given over the telephone, and that at the time of the test an appointment should be made to return for the test results. For other STDs, practice will vary, but in no circumstances should results be released without verification of adequate identification. When seeing the patient the practitioner should have in front of him or her the notes of the pre-test counselling and proceed on the basis of both these and the test results. Essentially, results will be either positive or negative (for HIV, positive on a screening test such as ELISA and positive on a confirmatory test such as Western blot). Unconfirmed positives should not be provided given the possibility, albeit very small, of false positives. In the rare case of indeterminate results, the result should be treated as positive until proven otherwise. Post-test counselling can conveniently be divided into counselling of people with positive or negative results.

Post-test counselling for negative results

Such counselling, provided that pre-test counselling has been adequately carried out, need not be time-consuming. The principal purpose of the post-test counselling session is to convey the results and to ensure that the person's prevention plan is being implemented. It has to take into account that a negative result may be taken as a 'licence to fly', and therefore the message that it takes only one incident of unsafe behavior to infect the person must be the first and foremost one given. The second purpose of post-test counselling for negative results is to reiterate information on how the virus is transmitted. Unless there has been any indication of failure to grasp the information in the pre-test counselling session, this can be in the form of briefly going over what is 'safe' in the way of sex (no penetrative sex) or 'safer' (penetrative sex using a condom). In the case of genital herpes, this will include specific instructions on the risk of transmission even when vesicles or ulceration are not present. In the case of injecting drugs, unused injecting equipment is 'safe' from the point of HIV transmission; cleaning with bleach, disinfectant or alcohol (two pre-rinses, two rinses in bleach, two cleaning rinses) is 'safer'. It is important to make clear the difference between 'safe' and 'safer'. 'Safe' means that there is no chance of transmitting HIV or herpes. 'Safer' means that the chance is reduced but that accidents (such as condom breakage, improper application, or inadequate cleaning of injecting equipment) can still not be ruled out.

If the patient has had repeated tests, it is advisable to clarify why. Many persons at risk have adopted health recommendations to both practise safer sex and to receive regular STD and HIV checks. These people typically deny any new risk behavior (beyond unprotected oral sex) in the period since the last test, and may be considered conscientious, informed, low-risk, repeat testers. A second group are those who report risk behavior despite previous education and testing. In this circumstance, the health provider should review the client's prevention plan, and where no realistic plan exists, consider the possibility that significant mental and/or sexual health co-factors are placing the client at risk. Appropriate referral can then be arranged. A third group presenting for repeated testing in the absence of reported risk behaviors include the AIDS phobic and compulsive, which should be addressed. Finally, the post-test counselling session provides an opportunity for the patient to clarify any matters that might have been raised and not completely understood or answered in the pre-test counselling session, or which have arisen since and require clarification.

Post-test counselling for positive results

This presents one of the most difficult situations for both practitioner and patient. It may have ramifications in clinical and psychological terms far beyond the initial fact of HIV or genital herpes infection, and the practitioner will probably have to deal at least with the immediate manifestations of these. On the other hand, if the pre-test counselling has been carried out, the process of conveying a positive result will be resting on a solid foundation. The practitioner will already know what chance the patient thinks he or she has of being infected and how the patient anticipates dealing with a positive result, as well as having some idea of previous coping mechanisms and supports. The pre-test counselling has been designed to make post-test counselling as well informed and appropriate as possible, and has set the stage in an interpersonal sense for practitioner and patient to have some sort of clinical relationship.

Advising a patient of results

Because of the trauma associated with positive results, adequate time (a minimum of half an hour, preferably more) should be allocated. Positive results should not be given on the telephone or on a walk-in, walk-out basis. Such a method of telling patients reinforces the idea that they are 'lepers' and makes it difficult if not impossible for the practitioner to make an assessment of the patient's mental state or need for further support or services. If the result is not expected by the patient, then the news is likely to be even more psychologically traumatizing.

Does the patient want to know?

In rare cases, patients may have decided that they don't want to know, and this should be respected. Normally, in this situation, the patient does not appear for the test results. Some patients may also wish to talk further about the issue before deciding to ask for the result. In all cases, it's useful to check by opening with a statement like, 'So you're here to get your HIV test results'. The patient can then confirm or disconfirm this.

Breaking the news

There is no easy way to break the news, and this section concentrates on the situation of HIV infection. However, the responses to news of herpes infection and counselling will follow the same pattern. If the practitioner prevaricates, or prefaces the news with a statement about how HIV infection doesn't necessarily lead to AIDS, he or she has already given the news, and in addition the information that the practitioner has trouble coping with it. The result is to make the patient feel that if the practitioner has trouble coping with it, how can the patient be expected to manage?

The issue of giving positive HIV results has been dealt with in some detail by Green and McCreaner,[13] and readers wanting to look at scenarios and role-plays of post-test counselling should refer to this book. Essentially, Green and McCreaner state that it is best to tell the patient straightforwardly, without evasion or qualification, what the results are. Any evasion or qualification may confuse the patient to the point where he or she is unsure exactly what the results are. Thus the post-test counselling starts with the facts (that the test result is positive, and that the patient has been infected with HIV, the virus that may cause AIDS).

Focussing on the response

At this point, there is a tendency for the practitioner to launch into explanations or qualifications. Don't. First, the patient may be in a state of shock and will not be able to take in much of what you are saying. Second, we are doing post-test counselling for the benefit of the patient's psychological state as much as for information. The next step is to focus on the patient's response by making a statement in the form of a question such as 'You seem quite surprised: did you expect this?', or 'This seems to come as a real shock to you', or even 'I guess that this raises a lot of new issues for you'. These questions give patients the opportunity to tell you *what* issues are immediate and uppermost in their mind, and in what order they want to cope with things. This gives the practitioner clues as to where to proceed on the *patient's* agenda.

Coping with the news

The reactions of people to the news will vary considerably. Responses will range from relief at having what was suspected confirmed, through to denial or inability to handle the information. It is important to let the patient describe his or her response and set the direction of the consultation. Green and McCreaner report that responses tend to fall into three main categories.

First, the patient may make statements such as comments of confirmation or denial of the possibility. The practitioner should indicate that he or she is listening and encourage the patient to go on.

Second, there may be reactions like silence or tears. There is a temptation to fill in difficult moments with talk. Avoid this: instead, if there is silence, ask patients to verbalize their thoughts (there may be many things going through their minds) as this will help the practitioner to determine what the central problems are. If the patient cries, again resist the temptation to distract or talk yourself. Seek clarification when appropriate by asking a question like 'What do you find most upsetting about the result?'.

The third response is a question. This may range from a factual question to a rhetorical one such as 'How will I tell . . . ?'. By posing these latter questions, which cover such areas as what he or she will do, and how the person will organize daily existence around his or her HIV serostatus (or herpes infection), the patient is not actually asking the practitioner for an answer. Green and McCreaner suggest that the questions are an invitation to discuss the issue from a number of different angles. Reflecting back the question ('You're worried about how X will react?' or 'How do you think that will affect them?') is probably the best way of starting the discussion.

Most common mistakes

On talking with patients about how they would prefer to be told, and about what actually went wrong with the way they were given their results, we found a number of common mistakes emerged. The most common is information overload. The patient is often sitting in a state of shock or contemplation and the session is filled with the practitioner talking. In a state of anxiety, the patient will either take little in, or worse, get the information muddled or wrong because he or she is only partially attending. Until you cope with the psychological reaction, it is pointless to give a lecture on the meaning of the result.

A second common mistake is for the practitioner not to provide the patient with the time and opportunity to come to terms with the information at his or her own pace. It is important to *follow up* with patients, to give them a chance to ask the many questions they will certainly have after the interview, or even just to provide an opportunity to talk about the situation later in a more prepared fashion. The worst thing the practitioner can do is to give the result and then leave the patient to his or her own devices. At a minimum, a further appointment should be made, and the patient given either an after-hours number with the invitation to call when in need of reassurance or information, or the number of an AIDS Hotline or information service. Don't leave the patient without a lifeline.

The third common mistake is to be too technical. Most patients will not have degrees in medical or biological science, so tailor your provision of information to their level. It is not uncommon to have patients complain that they didn't understand a word of what they were told by a practitioner because it was so technical. Even the term 'positive' is confusing to the medically unsophisticated, and concepts such as latency, defence systems and germs may be too much for some patients. The message is simple—therefore keep it that way, and encourage questions so that patients can learn more if they want to, and so that you can get an idea of what they really understand.

Discussing the issues

There will be a number of issues raised by the patient which need to be discussed. These will include several mandatory pieces of information. First, it must be made clear that in the case of HIV infection, being infected does not mean that the patient will necessarily go on to have fully developed AIDS, and that HIV infection is not the same thing as AIDS. Of course, if the patient shows signs or symptoms of AIDS, it would not be appropriate to raise this issue. Second, the issue of who should be told must be raised. It is not uncommon for patients to be so distraught as to tell people who, on reflection, are inappropriate, and this may often lead to the information being widely and indiscriminately spread. Alternatively, it may also lead to discrimination and rejection. Because the patient will want to confide in and receive support from significant others, this issue should be raised and social support mechanisms assessed.

At this stage, the practitioner is making an assessment as to whether the psychological response is appropriate or whether there may be additional issues arising. If patients have a history of depression, suicide attempts, or have indicated in pre-test counselling that this is something they have considered, referral for psychiatric assessment—and until this occurs, close monitoring—is mandatory. In cases such as this it may be wise to give the patient the practitioner's after-hours number or to advise the locum or covering practitioner of the situation.

One of the central issues in the discussion (which may cover more than one session) is coping with the diagnosis. When the patient raises such issues the practitioner, rather than focussing on the inability to cope, should try to make a list of the problems foreseen. Then go down the list and take the problem that appears to be most amenable to solution, and elicit from the patient the possibilities for managing the issue. In the first session, if there is time, try to cover only one or two, and leave others until later sessions if possible to avoid overload.

Remember that if the patient is shocked by the test result she or he will tend to see things fairly negatively, and thus attempting to force concentration on issues of coping (particularly when it may take some time for the news to sink in) is inappropriate. These matters should be dealt with as raised by the patient (possibly with some gentle encouragement) and not laid on the person when he or she may be unable to cope with them.

The advent of new treatments for HIV, and early aggressive treatment to reduce viral load, raises the question of how soon following provision of the test results to commence treatment. Physicians may wish to take further blood samples to establish viral load baselines, and may feel a tension between this and respecting the time the person needs to adjust to being positive. It's important in this circumstance that the physician considers each individual's reaction and develops an appropriate plan for follow-up. While a blood draw at post-test is now common practice, complex review of treatment options and initiation of treatment regimens are best left for a follow-up session.

Finally, patients in early stages of adjustment to HIV disease may request a life prognosis. There is no reason at all that a person with HIV or genital herpes infection cannot lead a normal life and have a reasonable life expectancy after infection. This should be emphasized, and you should encourage the patient to see the question as being one of life continuing rather than ending. Even in the most difficult situation, don't take all hope away from the patient.

Concluding the session

Reassurance that the practitioner will continue to assist the patient, confirmation of a follow-up appointment or referral to a specialist to discuss treatment, and expression of personal support are three important aspects to convey at the end of the consultation. While this may be taken for granted by the clinician, there are enough stories, both true and apocryphal, of perceived rejection of patients by practitioners, to make this mandatory (for both HIV and herpes). Patients have described in graphic terms the trauma

145

of receiving a positive result from an HIV test[14] or genital herpes test,[15] and thus the follow-up appointment within the next few days is essential.

Issues for a later session

Because AIDS is a high-profile epidemic (as herpes was in the early 1980s), unlike the case with other infections, patients may be quite well informed through the media and confronted variously with pessimistic morbidity and mortality statistics and/or promises of cure. While health practitioners are often asked for precise information on the likelihood and timing of disease progression in the case of HIV, we believe it is neither helpful nor accurate to make predictions. Such information is unlikely to be of benefit to the patient and may encourage a sense of fatalism or despair. Where patients' prognosis is poor—as in situations of advanced HIV disease—it is important not to remove all hope.

There are a number of other issues that should be addressed at a subsequent session. These include information about the disease, treatment options, discussion of the implications of the disease (on mental health, relationships, sexual response, having children, life insurance, work, stigmatization, health care and vaccinations) and prevention of transmission.

At the first follow-up session, it is important to clarify patients' understanding of what being HIV positive means. Do they understand that they are infected and can transmit this infection to others? A natural opportunity exists to ask them how they have coped with the news, and what follow-up questions they may have. In this way, the physician can assess the degree of adjustment following diagnosis.

The complex treatment regimens currently available to treat HIV require good adherence. For this reason, it is important to assess if the client is stable enough to discuss treatment options and to discuss long-term implications of starting on various regimens. Patients who state that they are too confused, or defer to the practitioner to decide, are probably not ready to manage and sustain a complex regimen of multiple drugs. Decisions not to initiate treatment need also to be respected. Throughout the post-test and early follow-up sessions, the physician has multiple opportunities to advance or hinder the empowerment approach to patient care (see chapter 7).

The patient with HIV infection should be warned of any symptoms that may indicate opportunistic infection, and be encouraged to seek a medical opinion if these occur. However, it is important to make this matter of fact and simple, otherwise you are only encouraging hypochondriasis or excessive preoccupation with bodily symptoms.

One of the important concerns of people with HIV infection is an apparent lack of control over disease progression (and with herpes, control over disease expression). This must be addressed for both physical and psychological reasons.[16] From the physical point of view, there are a number of drug trials available, and they should be discussed with the patient. Disease progression or expression can probably be influenced by sensible diet, exercise and looking after oneself. Reduction of stress and adequate relaxation are also factors that may slow progression of disease, particularly in the case of herpes. Thus, even in the absence of commencing aggressive treatment, there are a number of options that patients can take to empower themselves, to maintain their health and possibly to slow disease progression or expression.

There are also a number of more traditional complementary therapies which should not be discouraged if they do no harm. These can have powerful benefit in helping the person to take charge of the disease, to maintain a hopeful yet realistic approach to living with HIV and to maintain both mental and physical health.

If patients are going to become anxious, depressed or suicidal, it is not uncommon for this to occur in the first days or weeks following a positive result. If this is explained to the patient, and the possibility of distress acknowledged, it makes it easier for the patient to make contact before an extreme situation develops. At the psychological level, control can be encouraged by discussing with the patient the things that are likely to trigger anxiety or depression, and suggesting that the person should try to avoid such situations if possible. Awareness of the onset of depression should be encouraged, and the patient urged to seek help if there are changes to sleep patterns, appetite, or increasing helplessness or hopelessness. Most depressive illnesses and anxiety states can be easily treated, and there is no reason why people should be condemned to misery or disease where amelioration is available. Given the possibility of psychological disease in people with HIV infection, it should be made clear that this is not something that has to be borne but that treatment for this should be sought and given, just as physical symptoms should be recognized and attended to.

At various points during early HIV care, it is important to address primary prevention of passing HIV on to others. The individualized prevention plan discussed at pre-test can be reviewed, and modified as necessary. Where a patient reports absence or loss of libido (both desire for and interest in sex), reassurance should be provided that this is common, and that it normally 'returns in its own time'. Traditionally, primary prevention has focussed on the prevention of transmission to HIV negative others. Transmission of multi-drug-resistant strains of HIV has now been demonstrated. Educating the patient that it is just as important for her or him to practise safer sex with HIV positive and HIV negative partners is essential. In addition to providing basic education, it is important to develop a relationship where the patient feels comfortable in raising sexual concerns. Where HIV positive patients are unwilling or unable to successfully follow risk-reduction guidelines, appropriate referral is necessary.

Referral

If the practitioner is not prepared or not competent to care for the patient, the patient will need to be referred to a specialist or clinic for immunological work-up. The patient may see this as a rejection because of his or her HIV or genital herpes status, so it is important to make it clear that this referral is for specialist attention and not because the practitioner can't cope with an HIV seropositive or herpes infected patient. Unfortunately, nearly one quarter of medical and dental practitioners surveyed in Australia said they would not be prepared to treat an HIV seropositive patient, so the fears of the patient may be realistic.

Where there are psychological sequelae or previous or concurrent psychological disturbance, psychiatric referral, or referral to a clinic with psychological services, should also occur unless the practitioner is comfortable and competent in dealing with psychological illness or maladjustment.

In summary, if the patient is HIV seropositive or has genital herpes, post-test counselling may appear to be one of the most difficult consultations for both practitioner and patient. However, there are a number of common issues that arise and the session usually follows a distinct form. If the practitioner bears this in mind and follows these guidelines, much of the discomfort and difficulty should be avoided and the session will benefit the patient and her or his response to the infection. The key to appropriate post-test counselling is to attend to the psychological issues before attending to the informational ones, and to take your cues from the patient as to the amount of time that will need to be devoted to each issue.

CONCLUSION

These guidelines outline the role of the general practitioner (and other medical specialists who may become involved in HIV or herpes testing) in making a clinical judgment on the appropriateness of testing; the conduct of pre- and post-test counselling; and some of the medical, psychosocial and medicolegal issues involved. It is important to note that HIV testing may have both positive and negative outcomes in terms of both the individual and the spread of the disease, and there is an obligation to assess each applicant for testing to determine whether the test is appropriate.

The role of the health practitioner is central in dealing with HIV and genital herpes infection. The medical practitioner will frequently be the first point of contact for those anxious about HIV or herpes and for those wanting a test for evidence of HIV infection, and can play a major and most productive part in preventive medicine. In the support and routine medical care of those who are infected, the general practitioner will again play one of the most important roles in the management of HIV infection and herpes, as well as many other sexually transmissible diseases.

REFERENCES

1. Goldmeier, D., Johnson, A., Byrne, M. and Barton, S. Psychosocial implications of recurrent genital herpes simplex virus infection. *Genitourinary Medicine*, 1988; 64: 327–330.

2. Ross, M.W. and Rosser, B.R.S. Counselling issues in AIDS-related syndromes: a review. *Patient Education and Counselling*, 1988; 11: 17–28.

3. Spencer, J. and Grey, J. AIDS: two case histories. *Australian Family Physician*, 1986; 15(1): 36–38.

4. Ross, M.W. AIDS phobias: a report of four cases. *Psychopathology* 1988; 21: 26–30.

5. Ross, M.W. Social and behavioral aspects of male homosexual behavior. In Coney, T.G. and Ward, T.T. (eds) *AIDS and other medical problems in the male homosexual.* Philadelphia: W.B. Saunders, 1986.

6. Kinsey, A.C., Pomeroy, W.B. and Martin, C.E. *Sexual behavior in the human male.* Philadelphia: W.B. Saunders, 1948.

7. Fischl, M.A., Dickinson, G.M., Scott, G.B., Klimas, N., Fletcher, M.A. and Parks, W. Evaluation of heterosexual partners, children and household contacts of adults with AIDS. *Journal of the American Medical Association*, 1987; 257: 640–644.

8. Bell, J. The thin latex line against disease. *New Scientist*, 1987; 154: 58.

9. Rosser, B.R.S. *Male homosexual behavior and the effects of AIDS education: A study of behavior and safer sex in New Zealand and South Australia.* New York: Praeger, 1991.

10. Dunn, K. and Leeton, J. *Birth control.* Melbourne: Pitman, 1982.

11. Ross, M.W. The relationship of combinations of AIDS counselling and testing to safer sex and condom use in homosexual men. *Community Health Studies*, 1988; 12: 322–327.

12. Cohen, M.A. and Weisman, H.W. A biopsychosocial approach to AIDS. *Psychosomatics*, 1986; 27: 245–255.

13. Green, J. and McCreaner, A. Post-test counselling. In Green, J. and McCreaner, A. (eds) *Counselling in HIV infection and AIDS.* Oxford: Blackwell, 1989: 28–68.

14. Richards, T. Don't tell me on a Friday. *British Medical Journal,* 1986; 292: 943–45.

15. Drob, S., Loemer, M. and Lifshutz, H. Genital herpes: the psychological consequences. *British Journal of Medical Psychology,* 1985: 307–315.

16. Macgregor, J. *Herpes: the latest word.* Melbourne: Currey O'Neil, 1983.

12 *Legal and ethical considerations*

Perhaps no other area of medicine requires greater professionality, attention to ethics, and patient sensitivity than sexual medicine. Schover and Jensen[1] outline professional issues that are likely to arise when the medical practitioner takes sexual histories and provides sexual counselling.

CONFIDENTIALITY

While confidentiality is necessary in all medical practice, it is of paramount importance when matters of an intensely personal and private nature are discussed. You need to make every effort to ensure that information about sexuality is shared by the practitioner and patient alone.

Schover and Jensen suggest that practitioners working in an institutional setting seek special permission to keep private notes only on sexual matters. Ward and outpatient notes are of necessity easily accessible to a wide range of health professionals and health professional students. We would suggest that it is perhaps just as important in the general practice setting, where notes may be accessible to non-professional persons. Especially in a country setting, it is quite possible that secretaries and receptionists will know patients socially. A second sensible practice is to question how much detail it will be in the patient's interest to record in the notes. For example, in taking a sexual history, succinct summaries may be more appropriate than detailed accounts, especially in situations like difficult divorces and criminal evaluations where the professional suspects the record may be subpoenaed.

Confidentiality in couples therapy is especially challenging. Even when a couple are being seen in joint therapy, separate files should be kept for each partner. The health professional is not at liberty to disclose information gathered in an individual session to anyone else without the written permission of the patient, including the other partner. When treating a couple both in individual and couples sessions, the professional should clearly establish the boundaries (in individual sessions with each partner) at the outset of therapy. If at all possible, the patient's permission—or in the case of couples therapy *both* patients' permission—should be sought before the case is discussed with colleagues.

THE SEDUCTIVE PATIENT

In any doctor–patient setting, the potential exists for the patient to behave seductively. Research suggests that a proportion of medical practitioners make positive responses to sexual advances. Some even claim that in psychiatric practice it may be therapeutic.[2] We take the stand that sexual intercourse with patients represents an exploitation of the doctor–patient relationship and should simply never be allowed to occur. In some jurisdictions it is illegal. Registration boards similarly tend to frown on sexual relations with patients and ex-patients and may de-register the perpetrator.

What then should you do? Simply ignoring sexual innuendo or physical advances is unlikely to solve the problem. Box 12-1 gives an example of acknowledgment of the patient's advance, gentle rejection of it and a firm re-establishment of the doctor–patient relationship on a professional footing. Schover and Jensen give guidelines for handling seductive or acting-out patients. These are outlined in Box 12-2.

A further suggestion is to have a colleague present, even under the subterfuge of an observational learning exercise.

BOX 12-1
The seductive patient

First-year medical students watched a video vignette and were asked how they would respond. They saw a very attractive woman aged about 18, who had returned for a check-up on an infected foot. She looked, rather fiercely, directly at the camera and said, 'I don't know how to say this, but I really like you. I think you're great'.

An extremely good-looking male student, presumably well used to dealing with such advances, gave this response. 'It's really nice of you to say that. Thanks. Now let's have a look at that foot.'

This reply graciously acknowledges the advance, defuses it and then returns the consultation to a professional basis.

CONSENT

It is important to remember that the patient has every right to refuse to talk about sexuality. There are three defining characteristics of informed consent:

- The patient should be told sufficient details about what is being agreed to and any risks involved.
- The patient should be capable of understanding what he or she is told. (Capability is often defined in terms of age, intellectual capacity or psychiatric state.)
- The patient should not be coerced in any way into giving consent.

Perhaps the last characteristic is most important here. Even though the practitioner firmly believes that it is in the best interests of the patient to discuss sexuality, the practitioner must be ready to drop the topic at once if the patient shows reluctance. It is enough simply to have made it clear that sexuality is an OK topic and thereby leave the door open for discussion in the future if the patient sees fit.

HOW MUCH DO YOU NEED TO KNOW?

Patients may perceive questions about sexuality as voyeuristic, especially when they have presented for diagnosis or treatment of a physical illness.

BOX 12-2

Guidelines for treating seductive patients

- Try to understand the patient's motivation in making the advance.
- Try not to react angrily. This will severely damage the doctor–patient relationship.
- Explore the meaning of the advance to the patient in a counselling framework.
- Consult with senior colleagues if you feel out of your depth.
- When working with patients with a history of sexual aggression, make sure the consultation takes place where the assistance of other people is easily available.

Derived from: Schover, L.R and Jensen, S.B. *Sexuality and chronic illness. A comprehensive approach.* New York: The Guilford Press, 1988.

The 'normalizing' approach which states that many patients with that particular illness find they are having sexual problems (see chapter 5) may overcome the difficulty.

Nonetheless, it is essential that questions about sexuality be asked only where they are related to the patient's welfare rather than to the prurient curiosity of the practitioner.

ETHICAL ISSUES IN STDS

Almond[3] was talking with specific reference to AIDS when she characterized two different and often conflicting ideologies with regard to ethical issues in sexually transmissible diseases.

- *Civil liberties:* The right of the individual not to be subjected to potential discrimination because of public knowledge that he or she has a sexually transmitted disease.
- *Public health:* The right of the community to protection from the spread of sexually transmitted diseases.

Box 12-3 gives a case history where a doctor found herself in something of a dilemma resulting from the conflicting modes of action derived from these two positions.

BOX 12-3
A doctor's dilemma

Stephen is a 46-year-old homosexual man. He has never had a steady sexual relationship and his sexual activities have been with casual partners and pick-ups only.

In July 1985, he was diagnosed as HIV positive and was counselled about safe-sex practices. He attended only one of the three counselling appointments given to him.

In subsequent consultations he said that he usually practised safe sex except on a few occasions. This was 'not much'. He rejected zidovudine therapy in favor of herbal remedies.

Since 1973 he had been presenting to the STD clinic with a variety of STD-related and non-STD problems. Since 1982, when he presented with a severe episode of herpes zoster, some if not all of the presentations could be related to HIV infection.

He remained remarkably physically well and up to October 1990 suffered no notable weight loss despite significant reductions in T4 cells and T4:T8 ratio.

In July 1990, Kaposi's sarcoma was diagnosed on biopsy. When the biopsy specimen was being taken he asked, 'You don't think it's cancer, do you, doc?'. He was told that the biopsy was meant to find that out and he declined to ask further questions.

A colleague who visited Stephen some four weeks after the diagnosis of Kaposi's sarcoma found that he was planning a massive reorganization of his garden and a protracted overseas trip.

His doctor at the clinic felt that he was using denial as a coping mechanism for the following reasons:
- His reluctance to ask questions or discuss his condition
- His lack of curiosity about his condition
- His continued practice of occasional unsafe sex
- The unrealistic nature of his plans for the future
- His rejection of zidovudine therapy.

The question was whether to make attempts to break through that denial. This might have had the public health advantage of discouraging him from unsafe sexual practices. His denial was also possibly a factor in his rejection of the preferred medical treatment. On the other hand, it is impossible to predict the mental and physical consequences of breaking down denial, especially given rather limited information about his premorbid coping style.

From: Bassett, I. Personal communication. 1990.

Box 12-4 outlines a recent controversy where the issue of the rights of the individual versus those of the wider community is again highlighted.

Crisp[7] focusses specifically on situations where the doctor faces a moral dilemma between respecting the interests of the patient and those of the community. His examples include:

- The patient who refuses to give up high-risk behaviors
- The patient who has asked not to be told the results of HIV testing and who tests positive
- The HIV positive person who refuses to tell the sexual partner
- The doctor who wishes not to treat an HIV positive patient
- The possible use of blood samples taken to confirm a diagnosis of anaemia in an anonymous research program to collect statistics on HIV prevalence
- The HIV positive doctor who intends not to reveal the fact to patients.

BOX 12-4

Testosterone replacement in HIV+ men

Of HIV+ men who show diminished sexual interest and/or sexual dysfunction, 92% show a clear cut improvement in sexual interest, satisfaction and erectile functioning with testosterone replacement therapy. Sexual activity increased and the men reported that they perceived an enhanced quality of life and an increased sense of vitality[4].

Clearly, the individual benefits from this intervention

On the other hand, Fisher[5] argues strongly that it is irresponsible in terms of potential risk to others to increase the possibility of HIV transmission by an intervention which has the likelihood of increasing sexual activity in an infected group known to have a high rate of unprotected sex[6]. This is especially so when the intervention may be offered at a time when the individual is suffering from AIDS dementia complex or other cognitive impairment.

Crisp gives alternative courses of action that the practitioner might take, but concludes that it is the personal balance of importance of the two conflicting ideals that will determine the course taken.

LEGAL ISSUES

The legal aspects of taking a sexual history and sexual counselling must also be considered. While these may change across jurisdictions, there are a number of common elements that the practitioner must be aware of. These relate to the legal obligations of the practitioner to notify particular categories of diseases, to carry out counselling with regard to particular diseases, and to disclose particular matters to the authorities. Further, the practitioner should be aware of the legal complexities of assault, confidentiality and consent.

Notification of disease

In almost all jurisdictions, particular diseases are notifiable to the authorities (usually the department of health) to aid in establishing the range and magnitude of disease in the community. Invariably these diseases include sexually transmissible diseases (particularly HIV, gonorrhea, syphilis and chlamydia, although specifics will differ from jurisdiction to jurisdiction). If a proven case of disease is diagnosed, then this is usually notifiable by name and with other identifying details. In the case of presumptive disease that is treated without definitive proof (e.g., without laboratory confirmation) the situation is less clear-cut, and the practitioner should seek the advice of the local health department on the criteria necessary for notification. There are usually special forms for notification, and the information is held confidentially and does not go beyond the officer to whom it is notified.

Disclosure

Disclosure of information to a third party should always be confirmed by obtaining written consent from the patient (with the exception of those disclosures required by law). However, there may be a number of difficult situations in which this is not possible. For example, if the practitioner treats both spouses or partners and is aware that one has had sex outside the relationship, yet is forbidden to convey this information to the other partner, then this instruction must be followed.

This situation is complicated when the infection that has occurred is a potentially fatal one (e.g., HIV infection). The legal situation has been complicated by several cases in the United States in which it has been held that if a person is in danger (the classic case was of danger from a psychotic patient who had indicated their intent to kill someone), then the practitioner has a duty to warn the person in danger. Just how far this can be generalized is uncertain, as is its application outside the United States. Generally, the safest option is to assume that, in the absence of permission, the threat must be a major and immediate one before confidentiality can be broken. Disclosure raises a conflict between the duty of confidentiality and the duty to protect third parties against foreseeable transmission of disease or other harm. It must be realized that possible consequences of disclosure may include discrimination, stigmatization and ostracism. In the area of HIV infection, Landsell[8] comprehensively reviews the issues that arise and in particular the legal duties in various jurisdictions. She notes that conflicts may easily arise between the individual's right to privacy and the interest of public health, safety and welfare. In general, unless the danger is foreseeable and direct (i.e., there is a specific danger to a particular individual rather than a broadly anticipated one), disclosure is not justified. That is, confidentiality is the rule unless there are extremely compelling reasons otherwise. However, there are exceptions to this in the realm of the criminal law.

Criminal law

Where the patient has committed a crime or acknowledges being the victim of a crime, the practitioner may be required to report this to the appropriate authorities. In most jurisdictions, laws exist that specifically cover sexual abuse, sexual contact with a minor, and protection of the vulnerable. Because laws differ between jurisdictions, the first step for most professionals is to know the law. In situations where the practitioner suspects he or she may elicit such information, for example in taking a sexual history, it is ethical practice to warn patients of the limits of confidentiality prior to taking this history. Based on the first principle of medicine—to do no harm—it is incumbent on the health practitioner to know and follow the law *prior* to making a disclosure. Unfortunately, the law is seldom simple. For example, in several jurisdictions, a sex offender who admits abusing many minors but fails to disclose the name or identity of any particular victim has not triggered any necessity to report; however, the case of a minor who reports one act of abuse will require reporting. In the former situation, the ethical obligation on the professional is to maintain the patient's confidentiality, while in the latter, disclosure with or without permission is required. In practice, where you are not clear on reporting requirements, calling your professional board (of medicine, of psychology, etc.) and outlining the case hypothetically is the simplest way to clarify your legal obligations.

There is no recognition of confidentiality in situations where the law requires health professionals to report. Hence, the second step is to follow the law. However—similar to the situation of partner notification—to preserve the practitioner–patient relationship the practitioner may wish to ask whether the patient prefers disclosing the information personally (in the physician's presence) or whether he or she prefers the physician to report it.

A third situation that requires violation of patient confidentiality in most jurisdictions is when patients are an immediate serious threat to themselves or others. In such cases, the practitioner may be required to take reasonable steps to restrain the patient until the police arrive.

Similarly, when the courts require that the practitioner provide notes or other documents, then the practitioner is obliged to supply a copy of these (regardless of whether the patient has given permission or not). Note here the distinction made between the criminal law (which concerns matters that are crimes as defined in the criminal law) and the civil law (which concerns such matters as damages and contracts).

Improper conduct with patients

This area has both ethical (as already noted) and legal aspects. What is considered *unethical* may not necessarily be *illegal* (e.g., in some jurisdictions sexual contact with a consenting patient). However, examination of a patient (particularly a genital examination) may be considered an assault if there is not a clear assent for the examination to occur. It is useful to spell out beforehand what is proposed and what it will involve. Clearly, the boundary between examination and assault is nebulous and from time to time patients do take their practitioners to court charging assault: this is usually in regard to genital or breast examination. It is wise to make sure that there is at least some other staff member in the building (although not necessarily in the room) when carrying out a genital examination, and if in doubt it is useful to have another health practitioner present or close by.

The issue of obtaining consent for specific tests (the most obvious case being HIV tests) is more clouded. This depends on whether the practitioner has got a blanket approval for 'some tests' or whether the tests have been specified. In general, it is wise to specify the tests involved, and opinion is divided over whether taking a test such as an HIV test without permission may constitute an assault. In some jurisdictions, the law provides that HIV tests may not be done without counselling and thus carrying out a test without such counselling carries legal penalties.

We have already noted that sexual contact with a patient is considered unethical. If this does occur, it may provide grounds for a civil action against the practitioner by the spouse, or action to de-register the practitioner for improper conduct. Generally, registration boards, medical colleges and other professional societies take a dim view of such conduct and de-registration or withdrawal of a licence to practise, or some other censure, may result. Thus, unethical conduct, while not specifically illegal, may have legal consequences.

Seeking advice

Where you are in doubt, you should seek advice. Many situations regarding ethics and the law are complex and involve specific knowledge of statutes, and weighing up a number of arguments for and against particular actions. Unless immediate action is necessary or required, it is strongly advisable to at least confer with a senior colleague, and if possible to seek the advice of your professional or registering body. In many cases, the practitioner has to weigh up the legal and ethical issues, which will not necessarily be congruent. For example, if the issue of maintaining confidentiality seems to outweigh the legal requirement to notify a crime, or vice versa. In such cases, consultation with senior colleagues is mandatory and will frequently clarify the issue without involving the practitioner in contentious situations. When in any doubt, consult.

REFERENCES

1. Schover, L.R. and Jensen, S.B. *Sexuality and chronic illness. A comprehensive approach.* New York: The Guilford Press, 1988.
2. Cart, M. and Robinson, C.E. Fatal attraction: the ethical and clinical dilemma of patient-therapist sex. *Canadian Journal of Psychiatry,* 1990; 35: 122–127.
3. Almond, B. (ed.) *AIDS—a moral issue. The ethical, legal and social aspects.* London: Macmillan, 1990.
4. Wagner, G., Rabkin, J. and Rabkin, R. Effects of testosterone replacement therapy on sexual interest, function and behavior in HIV+ men. *Journal of Sexual Research,* 1997; 34: 27–33.
5. Fisher, W.A. Do no harm: on the ethics of testosterone replacement therapy for HIV+ persons. *Journal of Sexual Research,* 1997; 34: 35–38.
6. Fisher, J.D. and Fisher, W.A. Changing AIDS risk behaviour. *Psychological Bulletin,* 1992; 111: 455–474.
7. Crisp, R. *Autonomy, welfare and the treatment of AIDS.* In Almond, B. (ed.) *AIDS—a moral issue. The ethical, legal and social aspects.* London: Macmillan, 1990.
8. Landsell, G.T. AIDS, the law and civil liberties. *Medical Journal of Australia,* 1991; 154: 61–67.

13 Understanding and counselling sexual orientation concerns

Historically, the health care provided to sexual minorities has been less than adequate, partly because health providers did not receive adequate education to achieve an informed understanding of sexual orientation concerns; partly because of negative physician attitudes towards homosexuality; and partly because, until 1970, lesbian, gay and bisexual concerns were hidden and not well understood (see below). This chapter opens with a review of background information all health professionals should know regarding sexual orientation, then examines specific health concerns related to sexual orientation.

HISTORY OF MEDICAL ATTITUDES TOWARDS HOMOSEXUALITY

Those patients who indicate to their medical practitioner that they are gay or bisexual will do so for a variety of reasons; for example, because they wish to discuss the area with regard to sexual counselling,[1] because they believe that this information will aid medical management, or simply because they are 'out' and volunteer a demographic important to them— in a similar way to heterosexual patients who may mention they are married. The trend to be out to health professionals (among others) is a relatively recent social phenomenon, however. It has been encouraged by the gay pride movement in the 1970s and necessitated for gay and bisexual men because of HIV in the 1980s and 1990s.

In 1980, Dardick and Grady[2] found that less than 50% of openly gay men in the United States had told their primary health-care provider that they were gay. One must assume that for those covertly homosexual, the figure was even lower. In Australia, over 20% of gay men presenting with sexually transmissible diseases did not tell the attending practitioner that their infection was homosexually acquired.[3] Unfortunately, one of the reasons for this is that three quarters of a sample of 1000 doctors acknowledged that knowing a male patient was homosexual would adversely affect their medical management.[4] In 1980, 84% of American physicians surveyed agreed that homosexual patients hesitate to seek health care because of physician disapproval.[5]

In 1981, Davison and Friedman[6] found that when two groups of psychologists were given a case history of a male, and one of the groups was told incidentally that the patient was homosexual, most of the patient's problems were construed by that group in sexual terms, and the sexual aspect concentrated on. It would appear that emotional biases, usually activated by lack of reliable information, adversely affected both medical treatment and patient counselling. Thus, at least until recently, physician homonegativity appears to have impacted on the health care of homosexual persons. Shilts[7] identifies physician homonegativity as one of several factors that prevented health professionals from responding to the AIDS epidemic until it was too late. Such an indictment of physician neglect fuelling an epidemic must never be allowed to recur.

UNDERSTANDING SEXUAL ORIENTATION

Definitions

'Sexual orientation' refers to adult stable sexual attractions, desires, fantasies and expressions towards other adult men and women. As defined, the orientation of a person cannot be determined until emerging adulthood. (See chapter 14 for a discussion of sexual orientation in children and adolescents.) Psychologists distinguish sexual orientation from attractions towards children and adolescents (termed pedophilia and ephebophilia, respectively).

Our sexual orientation is only one aspect of our larger sexual identity. Other components include one's assignment at birth based upon one's external genitalia as being male and/or female; *gender identity*, one's sense of being a man and/or woman determined intrapsychically; and *social sex role*, one's masculinity and/or femininity as defined by society and cultural tradition.[8] Each aspect of identity appears relatively independent of the others. Thus, it should not be assumed that a masculine or androgynous female patient is attracted to women, or that a male who reports identifying as a woman (i.e., transgendered) is attracted to men.

Sexual orientation includes the gender(s) of those one finds erotic; the gender(s) of the person(s) on whom one's sexual thoughts focus, fantasies and desires; and the gender(s) of persons with whom one bonds emotionally and falls in love. Patients differ in the importance they ascribe to their sexual orientation, with some considering it incidental and others critical. Sexual orientation may help to define a patient's community, political and even spiritual identification(s).

Incidence of homosexuality

Is homosexuality normal? Statistical estimates of homosexuality vary widely, dependent in part on the definitions used. For example, using the Kinsey data, between 3% (current exclusive homosexual behavior and attractions) and 50% (any adult same-sex behavior, desire or fantasy) of Americans in his sample could be considered homosexual.[9]

Using a stratified population sampling technique in a national study of 2601 Australian adults, Ross[10] found 11% of men and 5% of women reported at least one same-sex adult sexual contact, 6% of men and 3% of women reporting it in the previous year.

A stratified national randomized study of 3432 Americans[11] aged 18–59 years found lower estimates: 3–5% of men and 1–4% of women reported some same-gender behavior (dependent on definition and time) and 3% of men and 1% of women reported some level of homosexual or bisexual identity. Because of social stigma, these should be considered conservative underestimates.

Homosexual behavior has been documented in all cultures studied, although the frequency and understanding of what constitutes homosexuality may vary markedly across cultures. Health practitioners working cross-culturally need to understand what 'homosexual' means in the patient's particular culture.

Together, these findings indicate that while most people experience their sexual attractions as being predominantly towards the other gender, some same-sex attractions and fantasies are a common part of human sexual experience. For a significant proportion of the human population, somewhere between 2% and 10%, a predominant to exclusive adult same-sexual attraction appears a normal part of human sexual diversity. Males and females may experience sexual orientation differently; specifically, men's attractions may be more innately determined, whereas women's attractions may be broader and, thus, more flexible.

Theories of etiology

In 1869, the term 'homosexual' was coined by the Hungarian scientist Carl Maria Benkert. Since that time, many different biological, psychological and sociological theories of the origins of homosexuality have been advanced. For a review of theories, we recommend you consult a textbook on human sexuality. While the precise causes of differences in sexual orientation remain somewhat speculative and elusive, what is clear is that no one factor causes someone to become homosexual or heterosexual.

No single scientific theory about what causes sexual orientation has been suitably substantiated. Studies to associate sexual orientation with genetic, hormonal, and environmental factors have so far been inconclusive. Sexual orientation is no longer considered to be one's conscious individual preference or choice, but is instead thought to be formed by a complicated network of social, cultural, biological, economic, and political factors.[12]

Myths and realities about homosexuality

Unfortunately, myths about homosexuality abound. Box 13-1 reviews some of these.

Homosexuality and mental health

Homosexuality is no more a sign of mental illness than heterosexuality is a sign of mental health. In 1957, Evelyn Hooker[13] published the first major study to compare the mental health of a non-clinical sample of homosexual and heterosexual men. Whereas clinical studies of hospitalized homosexual men found evidence of associated mental illness, her study found few differences in psychopathology. She concluded that the pathologization of homosexual orientation was without medical basis or justification. Based upon these and subsequent findings, in 1974 the American Psychiatric Association removed homosexuality as a pathological condition.

However, social stigma towards homosexuality has been demonstrated to have a negative impact on mental health. Ross's[14] four-country comparative study, and Rosser's[15] two-country comparison both found evidence of poorer adjustment in those countries that were more sexually conservative and homophobic. The results are consistent with the premise that homosexuality, in and of itself, is not related to psychological (mal)adjustment; rather the perpetuation of homophobia, prejudice and isolation within the wider society negatively impacts on mental health. This is further supported by recent research within a country comparing homosexual men with low and high degrees of internalized homophobia. Internalized homophobia appears to be associated with poorer mental and sexual health adjustment.[16]

BOX 13-1
Myths and realities of homosexuality

Myth	*Reality*
• Homosexuality is the result of abnormal parenting.	• Gays come from a wide variety of family backgrounds, both good and bad.
• Homosexuality is the result of incest or being sexually abused.	• Most gay men and lesbian women report no sexual contact with adults as children.
• Homosexuals prey on youth to maintain their lifestyle.	• Most pedophiles and ephebophiles identify as heterosexual men.
• A 'good woman/man' or getting married (heterosexually) cures homosexuality.	• Life stories of married gays and lesbians suggest heterosexual intercourse is not as satisfying, nor does it change one's sexual orientation.
• Gays/lesbians lead sad lives fraught with loneliness, self-hatred and meaningless relationships.	• Most gay and lesbian people report being happy and self-accepting, despite the difficulties of living in a non-accepting society.
• Gays/lesbians are a threat, to society offering little and selfishly using society for their own sordid ends.	• Lesbians and gays participate in society at all levels and generally make good citizens.

Derived from: Rosser, B.R.S. *Gay Catholics Down Under.* 1992.

Understanding the sexual orientation continuum

McConaghy[17] notes that both within gay subcultures and in wider society, seeing people as *either* gay *or* heterosexual is still the most common way people view orientation. This is particularly problematic for bisexual patients and those at early stages of exploring their sexual identity. A common mistake in counselling sexual orientation issues is to present sexual orientation as a dichotomy (people are either homosexual or heterosexual) or a trichotomy (gay/lesbian, bisexual or heterosexual). This overaccentuates differences and can lead to the patient feeling 'boxed in' by the practitioner. Kinsey[9] concluded that orientation fell on a continuum, from exclusive homosexuality at one end, to exclusive heterosexuality at the other. Further, he noted that some same-sex activity resulting in orgasm was relatively common in adulthood, and that people's orientation (measured by behavior and attraction) moved along this continuum over time and circumstance. While fewer men were found to be exclusively homosexual than exclusively heterosexual during the previous three years, and fewer women reported homosexual behaviors than men, Kinsey conceptualized that sexual orientation, like most other natural phenomena, was probably normally distributed across the homosexual–heterosexual continuum, attributing the differences in gender and orientation to social pressure and stigma.

Sexual orientation labels

Whereas 'homosexuality' had been coined by a doctor investigating deviance, the term 'gay' has come out of the gay movement as a description of homosexual subculture. It is a more positive and respectful term for someone self-identified and accepting of her or his homosexuality.

'Lesbian' derives from the community of women formed by the female poet Sappho, c. 600 BC, on the Greek island of Lesbos. As 'gay' and 'lesbian' have become the accepted identity labels, the term 'homosexual' is increasingly restricted to a description of same-sex behavior or attraction. When counselling patients, it is a good principle to take your cues from how they define themselves, and to use the patient's language in discussing sexual orientation concerns.

Development of sexual identity and sexual identification

Our sexual identity and adjustment do not develop in a vacuum, but are shaped by family, social and cultural understandings of what same-sex and opposite-sex attraction and behavior mean. Coleman[18] and Cass[19] have proposed paradigms of homosexual identity development which can assist the practitioner to assess and understand stages of 'coming out'. Both models stress the necessity for human beings to develop: in order to identify their dominant sexual orientation; to resolve the intrapsychic, interpersonal and social implications of their orientation identity; and to integrate their sexuality into their wider sense of self for healthy sexual and mental functioning. Failure to resolve questions of orientation risks infantilism of sexuality or reversion to an earlier stage with accompanying psychological distress and long-term negative impact on mental health.

Maturational theory, combined with the psychological studies cited above, suggests that many, if not most, people resolve their sexual orientation questions by coming to identify as homosexual/gay or heterosexual/straight (and some as bisexual), even if their internal attractions and desires are more complex than these labels acknoweldge. Both Coleman's and Cass's models stress the importance for mental health of people being able to experience their sexual orientation in a positive way.

Cass's model posits six stages in the development of a homosexual identity in the individual:

1. Identity confusion
2. Identity comparison
3. Identity tolerance
4. Identity acceptance
5. Identity pride
6. Identity synthesis.

Identity confusion describes the stage where individuals feel that they are different from others and that their feelings or behaviors may be labelled as homosexual. The second stage, identity comparison, is where the individual makes the first tentative commitment to a homosexual identity and the realization of being homosexual to a degree.

With identity tolerance in the individual comes the recognition that he or she is probably homosexual and a degree of commitment to this identity arises. By stage 4, the identity acceptance stage, the individual accepts the label of homosexual, at least in gay company, and begins to socialize within a gay subculture. The stage of identity pride is marked by wide disclosure and open activism and describes the situation where everything the individual does is defined primarily by his or her homosexuality. At this stage, the central identity of the person is as a homosexual.

The sixth stage of the Cass model is perhaps the one that has stimulated most debate. In the individual, the 'them versus us' view of homosexuals and heterosexuals fades, and is replaced by a situation where the person's homosexual identity is seen as being one of a series of identities, but not one that defines all aspects of the person's life. The individual may thus see being homosexual as an incidental matter like political belief or occupation, and not something that he or she is all the time. It is important that we deal with patients' sexuality depending on the level of acceptance they are at and do not try to push them too fast through these stages. We should let them achieve these stages, with encouragement, at their own pace.

Coleman has also developed stages of homosexual identity formation. His stages are as follows:

1. Pre coming-out
2. Coming out
3. Exploration and experimentation
4. First relationships
5. Integration.

Each stage of the coming out process raises unique health challenges both for the health provider and for the patient. Using Coleman's stages of coming out, Rosser[20] has identified clinical concerns associated with each stage of the process. During the first stage, 'pre coming-out', the predominant clinical concern is orientation distress. The patient may be seriously depressed and even suicidal. While coming out, intrapsychic and interpersonal conflicts emerge and dominate. During Coleman's third stage, exploration, it is important that the provider affirm the person's exploration of her or his sexuality, the challenge being to address safety issues including safer-sex counselling. Following this stage, first relationships emerge as the central preoccupation of the patient. Clinical issues of dependence, isolation and abandonment of safer-sex guidelines are prominent. Once integration is achieved, the major clinical concerns are unlikely to be related to the person's sexual orientation, except in situations of stress and/or trauma. In such situations, the major clinical concern becomes regression to earlier stages and conflicts.

Can sexual orientation be changed?

Freud noted that homosexual orientation appeared stable in most adults, resistant to modification through analysis, and benign. Reorientation therapies attempt to modify sexual orientation, typically from homosexual to heterosexual. The ethicist Murphy[21] notes that despite the myriad of twentieth century interventions that have attempted to modify homoerotic orientation (including chemical castration, neurosurgery, electroconvulsive shock treatment, incarceration, aversion therapy, heterosexual religious conversion and deliverance) not one case has been found where reorientation was convincingly demonstrated. While many of these techniques were able to demonstrate behavioral modification, none was able to change the deeper affectional orientation. Indeed, it is a testament to the resilience of human sexuality that despite the many techniques attempted, none have proved effective.

In recent years, the practice of attempting to help dysphoric homosexual patients impose a heterosexual orientation has declined significantly. Factors influencing this decline include the poor success rate of reorientation, the fact that homoeroticism is no longer considered pathological, the long-term negative effects reported by those who underwent reorientation therapy, and the serious ethical concerns raised by these attempts. The American Psychiatric Association, American Psychological Association and even the conservative American Medical Association all have condemned such practices as unethical, ineffective and harmful.

Some patients may ask your opinion about religious groups for 'ex-homosexuals'. Some conservative religious groups still provide 'deliverance ministries' to reorient people from homosexuality. Evidence from these groups suggests that where a person is highly motivated, strongly religious, highly diligent, has some pre-existing heterosexual desire, and remains within the religiosocial culture, some modification, at least short term, may be possible. Two studies have been undertaken demonstrating long-term modification in 3–5% of attendees. As this change rate approximates natural variation seen in longitudinal studies, critics argue the interventions are ineffective, and sometimes dangerous. In summary, it appears possible to make someone function heterosexually, but deeper markers of orientation such as attractions and the ability to fall in love appear to be more innate.

From the point of view of the general practitioner, it is important to be aware that patient requests to modify sexual orientation may reflect problems of stigma management and be symptomatic of difficulties more amenable to counselling, rather than to take the patient's request at face value. It is also necessary to differentiate a homosexual orientation from core or marginal transvestism or transsexualism. A few homosexuals may request gender reassignment in order to make their same-sex desires 'legitimate' by becoming a member of the 'opposite sex'.

COUNSELLING ISSUES RELATED TO SEXUAL ORIENTATION

There are some helpful tips to consider when discussing orientation with patients. Any time someone reveals something sexually personal, it is

---

BOX 13-2

A poor response to disclosure

One of us (LDC-L) was treating a 33-year-old single male actor for performance anxiety, which was severely affecting his ability to succeed at auditions.

During the third session, he revealed that he was gay.

'Oh yes, I realized that', was the blithe response.

The man was terribly distressed and wanted to know all the signs of behavior and appearance that made his homosexuality apparent. A lame mutter about lots of actors being gay did little to save the situation.

A much better response would have been to say, 'Ah yes. Now how do you feel this affects things?'.

---

important to realize that this decision has probably not been taken lightly. This holds for disclosure of sexual orientation and identity. It is helpful to remember that in the physician–patient interview, just as a practitioner may be assessing a patient, so the patient is assessing the practitioner. An understanding and accepting response is both important and appropriate (see Box 13-2). Because homosexuality is relatively common, it is particularly important not to assume that all patients are heterosexually oriented unless you are advised to the contrary. The use of gender-neutral terms (until clarified), and clearly distinguishing between behavior and identity, will prevent the practitioner from making obvious mistakes. Box 13-3 lists screening questions regarding sexual orientation concerns.

Homosexuality as a health concern

When a patient has revealed his or her homosexual orientation, there can be a tendency to understand this as pertaining only to sexual matters, which is a particularly narrow definition. While this information may mean examining additional sites for sexually transmissible diseases if the patient engages in receptive anal intercourse (anorectal as well as the usual urethral and oropharyngeal sites), it also has much wider implications.

It is important to assess how the patient feels about his or her sexual orientation, and in particular whether he or she is 'out' or 'closeted'. Being closeted has negative health implications. In terms of psychosomatic illness,

---

BOX 13-3

Screening questions concerning sexual orientation

- Are you currently sexual with males, females or both?
- In the past, have you been sexual with males, females or both?
- In terms of how you see yourself, what is your sexual orientation? (Probe: Do you identify more as gay, bisexual, straight, none of the above or something else?)

---

these can include unexplained headaches, hypertension, gastrointestinal disorders ranging from ulceration to irritable bowel syndrome, and asthma which has a functional component. Sexual orientation distress, (also referred to as 'ego-dystonic homosexuality', and 'internalized homophobia') is a significant mental health concern, and identified patients should be referred to appropriate health professionals for help. Psychological stress may also present in a variety of less somatic forms, such as sleep disturbance or generalized anxiety. In most cases the stress is manageable through an accepting clinical interaction or referral to stress management programs and relaxation training. In addition, the practitioner should consider referral to a mental health professional to address sexual acceptance issues.

The great majority of openly gay men, lesbian women and bisexual persons will experience few or no problems with their sexual orientation. Such patients may be remarkable in psychological terms only where stigma management presents as an issue. For this reason, most counselling related to sexual orientation, apart from general problems which face all individuals, relates to management of stigma.

HOMOSEXUAL RELATIONSHIPS

The popular view of the homosexual as single and promiscuous is not an accurate one for the great majority of gay individuals. A survey of gay men in the United States found that the median number of lifetime sexual partners of sexually continuously active individuals was less than 50.[22] It is important to bear this in mind when reading of atypical samples (e.g., many AIDS cases) in which sexual partners may number in the hundreds or thousands.

BOX 13-4

Questions to assist sexual orientation exploration

- What sort of person or person(s) are you most attracted to?
- What do you like most in a man/woman?
- If you could do anything to explore your sexual orientation, what would you like to do?
- What sort of homework exercises would be helpful for you to explore further your attractions and desires?
- What do you look for in a partner?
- What would it be like for you to tell your parent/spouse about these attractions?
- What do you like most about your sexual orientation?
- What things are hardest for you concerning your sexual orientation? (Probe: How bad did it get?)
- What would you do differently if you had just a little more belief in yourself, a little more courage, a little more trust?

Most gay men and lesbian women have at least one long-term significant relationship. As with heterosexual couples, a patient disclosing being in a committed relationship does not necessarily imply monogamy. Same-sex relationships have been classified into five general categories by Bell and Weinberg.[23] They divided their sample into:

1. Close-coupleds
2. Open-coupleds
3. Functionals
4. Dysfunctionals
5. Asexuals.

The 'close-coupleds' were closely bound together and monogamous, in the sense that the two individuals tended to look to one another for sexual and interpersonal satisfactions. They had the lowest level of sexual or psychological problems.

The 'open-coupleds' were living with a special sexual partner, but tended to seek sexual interpersonal satisfactions with people outside their partnership, although this tended to worry them. Psychologically and sexually, they had no more or less problems than other groups.

The 'functionals' were the equivalent of the swinging singles, and appeared to organize their life around their sexual experiences. They tended to have wide social circles and few sexual and psychological problems.

In contrast, the 'dysfunctionals' were troubled people whose life offered them little gratification and who displayed significantly greater psychological and sexual problems than any other group. This group most closely accorded with the old stereotype of the tormented homosexual.

While this sketch of homosexual relational patterns is brief, it does indicate the great diversity of interpersonal styles that exist within a homosexual lifestyle.

SEXUAL PRACTICES AND SEXUALLY TRANSMISSIBLE DISEASES

The practitioner cannot assume behavior and risk of STDs from a patient's identity. Almost all sexual activities are practised by both heterosexual and homosexual persons, with the exception of penovaginal intercourse in exclusively gay men and lesbian women. It is not generally realized that anal-receptive intercourse is practised regularly by one in twelve women,[24] while one third of homosexually active men report never engaging in anal sex.[15] While most human beings have preferred sexual activities, some men and women also prefer a particular role in same-sex situations (e.g., being the insertive or receptive partner) while others enjoy both roles, or different roles in different circumstances.

Contrary to popular opinion, anal intercourse only occurs in about one third of male homosexual encounters. Fellatio and mutual masturbation are more common in terms of frequency.[14] In female–female sex, activities will most commonly involve oral or manual stimulation.

From a medical point of view, anal intercourse if carried out with inadequate lubrication or any great degree of rigour may lead to lesions of the rectal epithelium which in places may be thin in contrast to the cornified vaginal epithelium. This may act as a portal for pathogens, and thus lead to greater risk than with penovaginal intercourse. From the sexual point of view, anodyspareunia (painful receptive anal intercourse) has only recently begun to be studied. Rosser and collegues[25] found that 12% of men who have sex with men report experience of anal intercourse where the pain was so severe they could not continue. Participants reported adequate lubrication, psychological preparedness (feeling relaxed and in control), and digital–rectal foreplay as the three most important factors influencing whether significant pain occurs.

STDS IN HOMOSEXUAL MEN

The range of sexually transmissible diseases in homosexual men includes HIV, syphilis, gonorrhea, non-gonococcal urethritis, hepatitis (A, B and C), herpes, and the so-called 'gay bowel syndrome' including infections, anal warts and proctitis.[26] While hepatitis and enteric infections are associated with analingus (rimming), a practice apparently much more common in the United States than in Australasia, it is important to note that the spectrum of sexually transmissible diseases is markedly broader in sexually active homosexual men than was traditionally assumed.

While the majority of homosexual men will not be at any greater risk of sexually related infections than heterosexual men, subgroups (those with multiple partners and a broader range of behaviors) are at increased risk.[27a,b] It is important to educate patients on appropriate prevention (e.g., hepatitis A and B vaccination) and test for additional pathogens in homosexually active men where symptoms occur. As an example, some 37% of Australasian homosexually active men may be surface antibody positive for hepatitis B.[27c]

Attitudes to sexuality and risk factors in homosexual men

A common error when dealing with patients (of any orientation) is to view the patient only in terms of specific diseases and disease risks. It is important to balance this tendency with recognizing and promoting the overall sexual health of the patient. For example, psychological and social factors influence sexually transmitted disease risk-taking.

Ross found that particular dimensions of sexual attitudes best predicted risk-taking.[14] These dimensions included attitudes to relationships, degree of control of sexual excitement and libido, degree of being visually stimulated by members of the same gender, social comfort, acceptance of one's homosexuality, and degree of permissiveness or prudishness. Homosexual men may vary across all of these dimensions. It would be a mistake to assume that the simple fact of a homosexual preference can predict anything about how the individual exists as a homosexual. Again, it must also be emphasized that the range of attitudes in homosexual men and women is as wide as the range of attitudes in heterosexual men and women.

Lesbian sexual health care

Lesbian women are at much less risk than heterosexual women of contracting sexually transmissible diseases[28a,b] and also enjoy on average much better mental health than heterosexual women.[29] They may still present with the same range of medical problems as other women, although these are unlikely to be directly related to their sexual preference. Most of the comments about sexual orientation health care apply more or less equally to gay male and lesbian patients. Lesbian women and female couples more commonly than gay men and male couples face additional issues of having children, and may wish to discuss options with their physician. There may also be greater difficulties with the management of social stigma, since lesbians face the possibility of double stigmatization (both sexism and homophobia).

COUNSELLING APPROACHES

When an individual wants to discuss his or her sexual orientation with their health practitioner, it is usually for one or two reasons. First, the person may want to give the practitioner information that may be necessary in health care (for diverse reasons, from transmission of sexually related diseases, to informing the practitioner that somebody the patient has lived with for 20 years is next of kin), and secondly, the person may want to raise specific issues or concerns related to his or her orientation. In many cases, the first disclosure will be to test the practitioner's response, and uncertainty or negativity usually preclude the matter being raised again.

Gentle inquiry as to whether being homosexual has caused any problems or special challenges may elicit further details if the patient is not forthcoming. For patients in the earliest stages of coming out, it should be borne in mind that the decision to reveal a homosexual orientation has usually been turned over in the mind numerous times, and that several visits may need to be made before an opportunity presents itself for the patient to discuss the matter. On the other hand, some patients will deny their sexual orientation if asked.

In many cases, the sexual orientation becomes the subject of concern, rather than the complaint about homosexuality being seen as symptomatic of other problems. For example, Serber and Keith[30] found that the reason their patients were dissatisfied with being homosexual and wanted to become heterosexual was because they were lonely and isolated. Following a course of training in social skills and assertiveness, the patients were able to interact socially with other gay people, and they reported that they were happy with their sexual orientation and no longer wanted to become heterosexuals (even if this were possible). Bell[31] comments in this regard that 'I am homosexual' is not self-explanatory, and such a declaration means different things to and about different people. Only after discussion by the patient of his or her position with respect to the various dimensions of homosexual experience can a more complete picture emerge.

It is helpful to clarify whether the patient's problems are intrapersonal (being unable to identify and function adequately as a gay, lesbian or bisexual individual), or are due to interpersonal problems brought on by being homosexual. This latter category includes negative reactions from family, employers or peers; marital or relationship difficulties; and in some jurisdictions where homosexual behavior is still proscribed, fear of legal charges.

COMING OUT: DISCLOSING SEXUAL ORIENTATION

'Coming out', as an individual's public acceptance of his or her homosexuality is known, is probably one of the most significant and potentially stressful moments in a lesbian or gay person's life. During this period, counselling may be sought, particularly as at this stage gay community support is not available or the person may feel too threatened to engage it. Often, the individual may not only feel that he or she is the 'only one in the world' but may also have no information about homosexuality apart from the myths and stereotypes. Hence educating patients that homosexuality is normal and recommending reading can be both helpful and reassuring.

Dismissing the patient's feelings as likely to pass is inaccurate and misleading, given that the person has usually become fairly certain over a period of several years that he or she is homosexual before confiding in others. Not infrequently, individuals at early stages of identification have trouble identifying their sexuality as homosexual because they do not fit the public stereotype (e.g., being effeminate), or because they also have some degree of heterosexual interest. Conversely, individuals may become anxious if they do not fit the conventional masculine or feminine stereotype, and counselling should follow a similar course.

Sometimes an individual will ask you if you think they should 'come out', or more specifically, come out to a particular individual (e.g., spouse, parent or friend). Because this is an area where different practitioners would provide totally conflicting recommendations based on their personal biases, we recommend that practitioners avoid giving advice. A better approach is to remain neutral, as in the interaction outlined in Box 13-5.

There are some other tips when assisting patients with sexual orientation concerns. First, it is essential to avoid value judgments about sexual orientation (positive or negative). Rather, affirming the person's honesty

---

BOX 13-5
Doctor, should I come out?

John was a priest in his forties who presented for help with sexual orientation concerns after suffering from a low-grade depression for many years. As he was trying to sort out his attractions to men, he asked his practitioner, 'Should I tell my parents and should I discuss this with my bishop? I'm just so tired of constantly having to hide who I am, and to pretend that everything's OK. It's not'.

The gay-identified practitioner responded, 'John, I don't know if you should tell your parents and bishop who you are or not. That's got to be your decision, and different people decide different things. What I do know is that it's healthy to be honest with yourself. Whether or not you come out to others, I think you do have to come out to you'.

---

and providing a safe place for the discussion of his or her concerns is recommended.

Second, information regarding homosexuality and the spectrum of sexual variation should be presented for the individual to be able to make his or her own assessment of who they are.

Third, provide permission for the patient to explore sexual orientation in safe and healthy ways (through reading, talking with knowledgeable friends, attending gay events and meeting places). The PLISSIT model,[32] outlined in earlier chapters, is a useful guide to assist practitioners to gauge level of intervention. Most general practitioners can provide permission, limited information and specific suggestions. Intensive therapy should be undertaken only by appropriately qualified specialists.

COMMON PROBLEMS

Common difficulties during the coming out process include reactions of family and peers that are negative (these sometimes may be resolved by counselling the family using the first two stages of the PLISSIT model), and the more complex problem of homosexuality within marriage. While this is a complicated subject[1] and cannot be treated in a generalized fashion, counselling should aim to define the degree of homosexuality and the point to which compromise is possible.

Similarly, it is often as difficult to advise on methods of counselling relationship difficulties in same-sex couples as it is to advise on the vast range of marital difficulties. What is essential is to determine whether the patient's homosexuality is bound up in the problem that requires counselling or whether the patient's homosexuality is essentially unrelated to it. The patient's sexuality should not become a central issue when it is not a cause of the problem.

In conclusion, successful counselling of sexual orientation concerns includes a lack of prejudgment, appreciation of the primacy of this issue to the patient, and sufficient knowledge of the area to provide accurate information and perspectives the patient may be lacking. While the counselling skills needed on the part of the practitioner are the same as those needed for other patients—genuineness, non-possessive warmth and accurate empathy[33]—it is important that the view of individuals as being *either* homosexual *or* heterosexual is not reinforced, and that the individuality of the patient is not submerged under this one aspect of his or her lifestyle. The ultimate goal of counselling should be to promote health; for patients to have an accurate and realistic acceptance of their sexual orientation, but not define their whole existence in terms of it.

GENDER DYSPHORIA, TRANSGENDER AND TRANSSEXUAL IDENTITY CONCERNS

Politically, transgender issues are often linked to lesbian, gay and bisexual issues; however, from the medical standpoint gender identity concerns are distinct from sexual orientations. 'Transgender', as an umbrella term, describes any cross-gender behavior, desires and identity. This includes everything from occasional cross-dressing in private to lifelong beliefs that one's natal gender is in conflict with one's gender identity. International standards of care for the treatment of transgenderism have been developed. These include regular counselling prior to hormonal therapy being introduced, and graduated stages of resolution of gender identity conflicts.

The treatment of transgender concerns is beyond the scope of this book, and requires specialist training in order to be competently undertaken. However, it is important for the practitioner to recognize and distinguish between sexual orientation and gender identity conflicts. Most patients presenting with gender identity concerns identify their sexual orientation as heterosexual, although cases of gender identity in gay and lesbian patients do also occur. Just as most gay men do not want to cross-dress, most transgendered individuals do not see themselves as engaging in same-sex relations. Issues common to both sexual orientation and gender identity conflicts include the need for acceptance, the need to access knowledgeable health care, the need to be open and honest with oneself (and usually others) about one's desires and identity, positive mental and sexual health promotion, resolution of social and familial conflicts, and assistance with dealing with a society that can be extremely unaccepting.

CONCLUSION

To summarize, while it is important to have a medical and psychological understanding of the range of problems common in sexual orientation concerns, it is also critical that we see these health problems as being neither solely sexually related nor stereotypically homosexual. In understanding and managing sexual orientation concerns, the central issue is to appreciate that homosexual individuals cover the same wide spectrum of humanity as heterosexual persons, and that the division of people into 'heterosexual' and 'homosexual' groups is arbitrary. The ultimate management mistake is to see patients in terms of their homosexuality alone and to ignore the fact that their sexual orientation may be a minor aspect of their identity and personality. The diversity of individuals who may be homosexual precludes generalization about them from the fact of their sexual orientation alone.

REFERENCES

1. Ross, M.W. *The married homosexual man: a psychological study.* London: Routledge and Kegan Paul, 1983.
2. Dardick, L. and Grady, D. Openness between gay persons and health professionals. *Annals of Internal Medicine*, 1980; 93: 115–119.
3. Ross, M.W. Attitudes of male homosexuals to venereal disease clinics. *Medical Journal of Australia*, 1981; 2: 670–671.
4. Pauly, I.B. and Goldstein, S. Physician's attitudes in treating homosexuals. *Medical Aspects of Human Sexuality*, 1970; 4: 26–45.
5. Sandholzer, T.A. Physician attitudes and other factors affecting the incidence of sexually transmitted diseases in homosexual men. *Journal of Homosexuality*, 1980; 5: 325–327.
6. Davison, G.C. and Friedman, S. Sexual orientation stereotype in the distortion of clinical judgement. *Journal of Homosexuality*, 1981; 6: 37–44.
7. Shilts, R. *And the band played on: Politics, people and the AIDS epidemic.* (2nd edn). New York: Viking Penguin, 1988.
8. Shively, M. and de Cecco, J. Components of sexual identity. *Journal of Homosexuality*, 1978; 3: 41–48.

9. Kinsey, A.C., Pomeroy, W.B. and Martin, C.E. *Sexual behavior in the human male.* Philadelphia: W.B. Saunders, 1948.

10. Ross, M.W. Prevalence of risk factors for human immunodeficiency virus infection in the Australian population. *Medical Journal of Australia,* 1988; 149: 363–365.

11. Laumann, E.O., Gagnon, J.H., Michael, R.T. and Michaels, S. *The social organization of sexuality: Sexual practices in the United States.* Chicago: University of Chicago Press, 1994.

12. Sex Information and Education Council of the U.S. (SIECUS). Fact sheet on Sexual Orientation, 1993.

13. Hooker, E. The adjustment of the overt homosexual. *Journal of Projective Psychology,* 1957; 21:18–31.

14. Ross, M.W. *Psychovenereology: personality and lifestyle factors in sexually transmitted diseases in homosexual men.* New York: Praeger, 1986.

15. Rosser, B.R.S. *Male homosexual behavior and the effects of AIDS education: A psychosexual study of behavior and safer sex in New Zealand and South Australia.* New York: Praeger.

16. Rosser, B.R.S., Bockting, W.O., Short, B.J. and Ross, M.W. Internalized homophobia and unsafe sex in men who have sex with men. *Abstracts of the 12th World AIDS Conference, Geneva, Switzerland,* 1998, June 18–July 3.

17. McConaghy, N. Homosexuality. *Sexual behavior: Problems and Management.* New York: Plenum, 1993.

18. Coleman, E. Development stages of the coming-out process. *American Behavioral Scientist,* 1974; 25: 469–482.

19. Cass, V.C. Homosexual identity formation: a theoretical model. *Journal of Homosexuality,* 1979; 4: 219–235.

20. Rosser, B.R.S. Clinical aspects of unsafe sexual behavior. *Sexuality Issues in Counseling and Therapy,* 1995; 1: 1–13.

21. Murphy, T.F. Redirecting sexual orientation: Techniques and justifications. *Journal of Sex Research,* 1992; 29: 501–503.

22. Darrow, W.W, Barrett, D., Jay, K. and Young, A. The gay report on sexually transmitted diseases. *American Journal of Public Health,* 1981; 71: 1004–1011.

23. Bell, A.P. and Weinberg, M.S. *Homosexualities: a study of diversity among men and women.* Melbourne: Macmillan, 1978.

24. Bolling, D.R. Prevalence, goals and complications of heterosexual anal intercourse in a gynaecologic population. *Journal of Reproductive Medicine,* 1977; 19: 120–124.

25. Rosser, B.R.S., Short, B.J., Thurmes, P.J. and Coleman, E. Anodyspareunia, the unacknowledged sexual dysfunction: A validation study of painful receptive anal intercourse and its psychosexual concomitants in homosexual men. *Journal of Sex and Marital Therapy,* 1998; 24: 281–292.

26. Ostrow, D.G. and Airman, N.L. Sexually transmitted diseases and homosexuality. *Journal of Sexually Transmitted Diseases,* 1981; 8: 75–76.

27a. Kingsley, L.A., Rinaldo, C.R., Lyter, D.W., Valdisseri, R.O., Belle, S.H. and

Ito, M. Sexual transmission efficiency of hepatitis B virus and human immunodeficiency virus among homosexual men. *JAMA*, 1990; 264: 230–234.

27b. Osella, A.R. Massa, M.A., Joekes, S., Blanch, N., Yacci, M.R., Cenzone, S. and Sileoni, S. Hepatitis B and C virus sexual transmission among homosexual men. *American Journal of Gastroenterology*, 1998; 93: 49–53.

27c. Burrell, C.J., Cameron, A.S., Hart, G., Melbourne, J. and Beal, R.W. Hepatitis B reservoirs and attack rates in an Australian community. *Medical Journal of Australia*, 1983; 2: 492–496.

28a. Lemp, G.F., Jones, M., Kellog, T.A., Nieri, G.N. Anderson, L., Withum, D and Katz, M. HIV seroprevalence and risk behaviours among lesbians and bisexual women in San Francisco and Berkeley, California. *American Journal of Public Health*, 1995; 85: 1549–1555.

28b. Bevier, P.J., Chiasson, M.A. Heffernan, R.T. and Castro, K.G. Women at a sexually transmitted disease clinic who reported same-sex contact: their HIV seroprevalence and risk behaviors. *American Journal of Public Health*, 1995; 85: 1366–1371.

29. Freedman, M. *Homosexuality and psychological functioning.* Belmont: Brooks/Cole, 1971.

30. Serber, M. and Keith, C.G. The Atascadero project: model of a sexual retraining program for incarcerated homosexual pedophiles. *Journal of Homosexuality*, 1974; 1: 87–97.

31. Bell, A.P. The homosexual as patient. In Green, R. (ed.) *Human sexuality: a health practitioner's text.* (2nd edn). Baltimore: Williams & Wilkins, 1979: 98–114.

32. Annon, J.S. *The behavioral treatment of sexual problems: brief therapy.* Honolulu: Enabling Systems, 1974.

33. Truax, C.B. and Carkhuff, R.R. *Toward effective counseling and psychotherapy: training and practice.* Chicago: Aldine, 1967.

14 *Sexual counselling of children and adolescents*

The sexual counselling of minors provides special challenges for health practitioners. Issues of language, of promoting normal development while not minimizing problems, of screening for sexual concerns while not unduly alarming minors, are all common challenges when counselling children about sex. In addition, the sexual counselling of minors and vulnerable adults raises ethical and legal issues regarding the patient's rights to health care and education on the one hand, and the parents' or guardians' rights to supervize information on the other.

TALKING TO CHILDREN ABOUT SEX

The principles for talking about sexual matters with patients as described in the previous chapters also apply when talking to children. Above all, it's important to be clear. When possible, use anatomically correct language (simplified as needed to aid understanding). Pictures should be used as needed, and the style of language should be factual, open and similar to that used for any other interview. Indeed, it is helpful to remember that the practitioner is often in a modelling situation: the child is likely to take cues from the practitioner on how to talk about sex (and may actually model language), how to feel when discussing sexual concerns (comfortable or not), and how in-depth the discussion of issues of sexual health should be.

There is no one correct time to raise or address sexual issues with minors. As for adults, when a child presents with illness or is in pain, sexual questioning is normally inappropriate (unless specifically related to diagnosis and treatment concerns). On the other hand, many health practitioners feel overwhelmed with the range of topics to cover during well-child examinations. Well-child examinations, however, are a natural opportunity to touch base with parents and child regarding sexual development and screening for sexual concerns. Box 14-1 summarizes questions to ask as part of well-child checks.

BOX 14-1

Screening questions as part of well-child checks

- Part of my role as your counsellor today is to check whether you have any other health concerns. I like to take this opportunity to review any sexual health concerns. Is that OK?
- How do you find out about sex? (Probes: school? peers? parents? church? literature?)
- Are you currently being sexual with anyone? (Probes: What sort of behaviors are you engaging in? What sort of protection are you using? Do you need condoms or anything else to protect yourself?)
- What sexual concerns are you and/or your friends dealing with?
- Many patients have concerns about their sexual feelings, their body, genital size, sexual attractions or behaviors that I might be able to help with. What questions would you like to ask about sex?

With all patients, but particularly with children and adolescents, it is helpful to consider the following hints for taking sexual histories:

- Use an open, positive, interested disposition when introducing sexual questions. Avoid two tendencies: dramatizing sexual health as somehow different from other areas and introducing sexual questions with statements indicating that parents and children have to be uncomfortable. For example, 'Many children find talking about sex embarrassing' can be intended to normalize an awkward silence; unfortunately, it also can send the message that children should be embarrassed about sex. Because children are frequently less conscious of and better able to articulate their feelings than adults, it can be easier just to directly ask the relevant questions.
- Start with other areas of health first, then weave sexual questions into the overall session.
- Gauge the child's communication ability by how they talk about other areas of health. The quiet child who doesn't respond to questions in other areas of health is unlikely to talk much when discussing sex. This doesn't mean the child has been abused or is shameful; it means the child is quiet.

- When doing physical examinations (e.g., of genitals and breasts), explain to the child *before* you examine her or him why you need to do this. Children who have been taught 'good touch, bad touch' rules, which include that no adult should be touching their genitals, need to understand that you are not violating the rules they have been taught to keep them safe.
- Goals in sexual assessments of children frequently need to be simplified. Children tend to give concrete answers to all questions, so the practitioner needs to be specific and to keep question content and construction simple.
- Remembering that there is no one perfect way to discuss sex with children can be helpful. Developing two or three different strategies is useful.
- The health practitioner plays an important role in promoting the healthy sexual development of the child. In particular, it is important not to pathologize sexual issues where the child doesn't recognize any or is not being harmed. In most situations, the practitioner is comparing the child's particular situation to formal or informal developmental norms. When thinking of norms, be mindful that these are averages; hence they include a diverse range of normal child activity. Many potential sexual problems can be avoided by reassuring parents that their child is somewhere in the normal range of childhood sexual development.
- At the other extreme, it is important not to dismiss or minimize a child's sexual issues. The girl who is worried there is something wrong because she doesn't look like her brother; the boy who is taunted at school by being called 'fag'; the child who is being molested; the pubescent child who is fearful because she or he does not understand what is happening to his or her body—all have serious issues that the health practitioner has an ethical obligation to address.

WHEN PARENTS HAVE CONCERNS

When the behavior is within the norm

Most sexual concerns of children come to the attention of the physician via parents. The most frequent concern parents raise is, 'Is my child normal?'. Many questions stem from parents' ignorance about childhood sexuality and sex play. In particular, some parents—especially those who come from conservative religious backgrounds and those with a history of abuse—may interpret the presumed 'innocence' of childhood to mean absence of any interest in sex or any activity that the parent may interpret as sexual. In the desire to protect their child, such parents are vulnerable to interpreting any sexual incident or interest as evidence of sexual abuse or a sexual problem. Hence, the first task of the physician is to establish who (parent or child), if anyone, has a problem. For most presenting concerns, assisting the parent in promoting the sexual health of the child is all that is required.

Children are sexual beings, and the tasks of childhood include sexual learning (e.g., of gender identity, social sex roles, body parts and functions). Unlike adults, most children have not yet learned to compartmentalize 'sex' as different from other learning. Hence, they learn through the ways open to them: self-discovery, play, reading, and by vicarious learning from and listening to other children and adults. When parents raise concerns about their child's normality, it is helpful to start by getting from them a brief summary of what is actually going on. If, in the health practitioner's opinion, the concern falls within the normal range of childhood exploration—masturbation, dressing up, playing 'doctors and nurses'—simple reassurance and education of the parents is the next step. Using the PLISSIT model, this is intervention at the levels of providing permission and limited information.

Two follow-up interventions can be helpful as part of preventive sexual health. First, referring the parent to a book about children's normal sexual development will reinforce your message, reassure the parents, and widen the scope of their education, thereby helping parents to recognize other situations as normal.

Second, it is important to assess the level of concern in the parents and to find out what sort of interventions they have already tried.

Punishment is seldom, if ever, appropriate in matters of sex. Because punishment for sexual activity in childhood may lead to sexual problems in adulthood, this should not be reinforced, and where punishment is already happening, the practitioner will need to intervene. Similarly, some parents will respond to a child's sexual activity by warning them to 'never to be caught doing X again'. Based on the sexual histories of hundreds of clients, this author is convinced that this intervention doesn't stop the activity; rather, it only drives the child into hiding the activity from adults and can increase a child's shame about sex.

A better approach is to view the child's development as representing natural opportunities to promote the child's sexual health. Unfortunately, many parents are likely to overreact when the child's issue has sexual implications, and many adults remain fearful of sexual education. The practitioner's role in such situations is to educate the parents about how to address the sexual concerns of their children in a positive and healthful way. Unless the behavior is physically harmful to the child (e.g., autoerotic asphyxia) or others (e.g., sexual molestation of younger children), assisting the parent to teach the child where and how to engage in this behavior appropriately is more beneficial. The principle here is that it is both more healthy and effective to modify a behavior to fit an appropriate context than to extinguish it.

Some examples may help. Young children's masturbation and self-genital touch is entirely normal, and parents should be educated to accept that. Showing a chart of children's normal stages of psychosexual development to the parent can be helpful. For older children, the parent can use the opportunity to teach a child that masturbation is a normal and healthy behavior, but something most people do in the privacy of their bedrooms. Rather than punishing a child for playing some version of 'doctors and nurses', parents can be taught to recognize the child's motivation. Once parents recognize that most childhood sex play is a child's attempt to learn about sex, the parent can then affirm the child's desire to learn by educating the child about gender differences and sex at an age-appropriate level. Similarly, the older child who likes cross-dressing can be encouraged to put on plays for the family, or to join a children's theatre company, which again normalizes the behavior, reducing shame and the child's feeling of being different.

When the behavior is problematic

A second level of intervention is appropriate when the parents' concerns appear legitimate: they either fear that their child may be experiencing harm and/or they suspect abnormal sexual development; for example, a child exhibiting a gender identity disorder; an effeminate boy or masculine girl getting harassed at school; or a child engaging in sex play that appears potentially harmful, or paraphilic. Here, the role of the practitioner is to assist both the child and the parent. In addition to soliciting a brief summary of the presenting concern, it is helpful to interview the parents alone to gain a more extensive sexual history. Box 14-2 outlines questions to ask in this interview.

It may also be necessary to seek confirmation about what is happening from the child. Usually, this is the easiest way of confirming or resolving parental or guardian concerns. Occasionally, however, it can be unhelpful or even potentially harmful. Hence, the practitioner needs to weigh carefully the pros and cons of counselling the child. Whether to have the parents present or absent during the interview should be the practitioner's decision, made in consultation with the parents, and eventually with the child.

In deciding whether to have a separate session with the child only, or a parent-and-child-together session, the interest of the child should be para-

---

BOX 14-2

Questions to ask parents when they have a concern about their child's sexual activity

- When did you first notice your child was doing X?
- Was there anything going on at that time that you think may help explain your child's behavior?
- Specifically, what is happening?
- How often is it currently happening?
- What is most concerning to you about this behavior, currently?
- What is most concerning to you about this behavior if it continues?
- What sort of things have you done to try and address this concern?
- Why do you think this is happening?

---

mount. For example, where the practitioner has established that a parent has already shamed a child for a particular behavior, a joint parent–child session is usually inappropriate until the parent's behavior has been addressed.

In a joint parent–child session, the practitioner should start by clarifying each person's role and the goal(s) of the session. An example of an opening statement is, 'Thanks everyone for coming in. How about we start by having someone summarize what's going on? By the way, in my office everyone has the right, if they're feeling uncomfortable, to say "slow down", "stop" or "pass", so we can go at everyone's pace and quietly get things sorted out'. During the first session, getting the parents' and the child's perspectives on the presenting concern (What is happening?), together with some history (When did it start? How has it changed over time?), goals (What they want from seeing you) and some diagnostic impressions, will probably be the most that is achieved.

It's important to go at the pace of the child. Many children take longer to verbalize, so set aside reasonable time for this interview. Use words the child can understand, be non-judgmental, and avoid taking any particular person's side. The role of the practitioner in such interviews is being a family counsellor: intervening between both parents and child to help all gain an appreciation for what is happening.

Consider the following tips for the beginning practitioner: the more anxiety he or she displays, often the more anxious the patient becomes, so it's important for practitioners to take care of themselves and know what they are about. For example, regarding many developmental issues—such as gender identity disorders, atypical social sex role, or sexual orientation concerns—the family may be very upset that little Johnny or little Sue is not acting the way they thought she or he would, but often there is no crisis. Unless you have reason to suspect that Johnny or Sue are in danger (e.g., from other children) or are a danger to themselves or to others, the primary role of the practitioner is (1) to reassure the parents that Johnny and Sue are normal and will develop in the fullness of time; (2) to help the parents face the reality that they may have a transgendered, effeminate/masculine, or lesbian/gay child; and (3) to assist the parents to continue to be loving guardians providing a secure and healthful environment in which their child can develop. With the child, the primary role of the practitioner is (1) to reassure the child that she or he is healthy and to monitor the health concerns (physical, mental, emotional) of the child; (2) to promote a healthy relationship between practitioner and patient, encouraging the child or adolescent that you are an available resource for them; and (3) where the child or others are in danger, to ensure the safety and welfare of the child. This includes referral to a specialist in children's psychological health as necessary.

SEX EDUCATION OF ADOLESCENTS

Adolescents remain at disproportionately high risk for HIV and other STDs. In the United States, one in four teens will contract an STD prior to adulthood. Many health practitioners are asked to provide sex education to adolescents either as part of their practice or in advising schools on curricula. Because sex education in schools has been a controversial topic, scientists have reviewed acceptable guidelines.

Abstinence promotion

Many health practitioners naively continue to promote abstinence as the 'safest form of STD prevention'. Since most people are sexually active prior to marriage and are at greatest risk of acquiring STDs during this time, practitioners should consider that, epidemiologically, this intervention has an unacceptably high failure rate. While abstinence (until marriage) promotion has been shown in some studies to delay onset of sexual activity for teens, once a person becomes sexually active it is neither appropriate nor effective. Advising abstinence to high-risk sexually active teens—and particularly for gay youth who cannot marry—tends to destroy the patient's trust and respect for practitioners who appear to be promoting a morality he or she is unwilling or unable to adopt. Hence, the American National Institutes of Health's consensus statement of scientists on 'Interventions to Prevent HIV Risk Behaviors'[1] recommends that where abstinence education is promoted, it is ethically necessary to include information on safer sex.

Safer sex promotion

Studies of adolescents show high rates of unprotected sex and STDs, and low rates of adolescent–health practitioner discussions about sex.[2–5] Only a minority of minors discuss HIV/STD prevention and condom use with their physician.[2–5] Yet teenagers who discuss HIV with their health practitioner are significantly more likely to use condoms and to receive education about condom use.[2,4] Most adolescents perceive their health practitioner to be the preferred source of information about sexual health related messages, including HIV and STD risk reduction. While 70–85% of adolescents in one study wanted information from their physician about HIV/STDs, condoms and sex, and wanted the physician to *initiate* the discussion, only 25% reported receiving any education.[4]

The problem does not seem to be a lack of perceived importance by practitioners. Studies of physicians[6,7] and recommendations of organizations of health practitioners internationally[8–16] have consistently recognized and encouraged more practitioner–adolescent risk-reduction discussions. Rather, the problem appears to be that practitioners and adolescents each prefer the other to initiate such discussions, resulting in a complicity of silence.

We believe strongly that similar to promotion of health in other areas, sexual health promotion, which includes education about safer sex, is an important area to prioritize in patient care. Assessing patients' knowledge of human sexuality, asking patients if they have questions about sex, and acting as a resource for sex education should be seen as part of the health practitioner's role in promoting overall health care.

Birth control

Related to the issue of safer sex is birth control and planned pregnancy. As with safer sex, the most natural time to discuss birth control is as part of a well-teen check and when a teenager presents alone or with a parent specifically requesting birth control. First, it is important to ensure the teenager feels safe to discuss honestly her sexual health concerns. While sometimes a teen may prefer her parent(s) to be present, most commonly this means inviting the parents to leave while you conduct the interview. It is usually easiest to start by finding out how much the teenager knows about sex, and then to discuss what sexual activity may be occurring. As with all patients, presenting some (but not an exhaustive list of) options, such as abstinence, condoms with spermicide, the pill and Depo-Provera, will be helpful for most teens. The most common mistakes are to assume the teenager is not sexually active, or that he or she knows more than he or she actually does. For example, one of the authors once treated a teenage mother of two children who was still uncertain where babies come from! Helpful approaches include inviting the teenager to ask questions, providing education and reinforcement for the teen for being responsible enough to seek consult ation, and outlining options that help the teen to be aware he or she has choices.

CHILDHOOD AND ADOLESCENT SEXUAL ABUSE

Current statistics estimate that one in four girls and one in nine boys will be sexually abused prior to becoming adults.[17] Most jurisdictions have specific laws that the health practitioner is required to follow when physical and/or sexual abuse of a minor is suspected or acknowledged. For example, any touching of the genitals of a minor by an adult (or a significantly older minor)—except in legitimate health circumstances—is illegal in most western countries, and the health practitioner is required to report the minor to the appropriate child protection authorities. Often such laws have been crafted to give clear and compelling guidance to the practitioner; for example, the practitioner *must* report regardless of how she or he obtained the information, the reason or rationalization given, and whether or not the patient provides consent. All health practitioners are required to be familiar with the laws of that particular area. The easiest way to do this is to contact the board of your professional organization and to request a copy of the ethical and legal requirements regarding sexual abuse.

Practitioners usually learn of sexual and/or physical abuse when the victim (or parent or guardian) brings it to their attention or when an offender self-discloses. Both situations require practitioners, first, to be attentive to ethical standards, especially to do no harm; and second, to understand the multiple roles they are required to play in this circumstance.

When a victim self-discloses

When a child or adolescent states that she or he has been abused, the first role or working principle for the health practitioner is to believe the patient.

Because shame and guilt frequently accompany sexual abuse and maintain the abuse dynamics when abuse is on-going, most minors are telling the truth when they disclose abuse. By believing the patient, and encouraging the patient to discuss further, the practitioner can also evaluate those small number of situations where a patient may not be telling the truth either because of mental health difficulties (principally delusional beliefs, paranoia and antisocial feelings) and/or secondary gain issues (when there is a clear benefit to the patient if the identified offender is investigated for offending). When a minor states he or she has been abused, the next step is to ask the patient, 'What happened?'. Throughout the process, it is important to go at the minor's pace, and to adopt a manner that expresses supportive, quiet concern. When a minor reports something that does not meet the criteria for abuse, this distinction can be clarified. When the self-disclosure meets the criteria, the practitioner can confirm that it sounds like abuse to him or her. When the practitioner is unsure, she or he can either ask for more information, or refer to a specialist to continue the interview.

Having been told about suspected sexual abuse, the health practitioner has an ethical, and often legal, obligation to investigate further. Especially in younger children, the assessment of suspected child abuse should be considered a specialist area of training. Again, the principal of 'do no harm' applies. Especially where a child may eventually be required to testify about the abuse, practitioners without advanced training in this area should refer to a pediatric specialist in abuse. This avoids having the child repeat the story more often than necessary, and avoids the risk, however unintentional, of leading questions contaminating evidence.

In the face of clear evidence of abuse, the practitioner's next step is to explain to the patient the proposed course of action. Informing the patient of what is happening and what needs to happen next is important—abuse by definition is the taking away of power from the patient by another. Hence, keeping the patient informed and appropriately providing them with options is crucial. Some patients may find it empowering to report the abuse to child protection; others may prefer the practitioner to do this. Either way, the practitioner should give the patient the option.

After the abuse is reported, two further steps are required. It's important to check that the patient is safe. For example, when a minor reports being molested by a parent, he or she should not be left in the unsupervized presence of that adult. And the minor cannot be returned home until the health practitioner is confident the alleged molester has been removed from the home. Second, the practitioner needs to think about the psychological and emotional safety of the minor. When minors blame themselves, they can be at significant risk of causing harm to themselves following disclosure. In situations of incest, the non-abusing parent—confronted with their spouse's actions, legal actions, and possibly withdrawal of family income— needs time to process the information, and to deal with her or his own feelings of blame. A stage of this process can include the parent blaming the minor for disclosing and even viewing the minor as an accomplice or seducer in the abuse.

Current theory and counselling on sexual abuse advocates strongly that the minor, no matter how provocative, is never to blame. The practitioner can assist the family in avoiding further harm by explaining such common reactions to the parent while assessing the environmental safety of the child. Whenever possible, the child's welfare and security must come first. Hence, even during assessment, the alleged offender is normally required to leave the home while the victim is encouraged to remain in familiar surroundings.

When an offender discloses

Sometimes the practitioner learns of abuse when the patient is the perpetrator (either an older minor or adult patient who discloses or has been found out). This situation raises complex conflicts of interest for the practitioner, including conflicting loyalties: the practitioner's first duty is always to the patient, and yet the law often requires practitioners to disclose to protect the victim, which may lead to negative consequences for the patient.

As always, the precept to 'do no harm' should remind the practitioner that even in the disturbing disclosures of molestation, the practitioner has an opportunity to communicate empathy and unconditional positive regard for the patient perpetrator. The adolescent who has been found molesting a younger sibling or other minors, exposing, voyeuring or engaging in other behavior legally defined as sex offending, normally doesn't have a clear understanding of her or his motivations, may be extremely frightened of her or his own behavior and what it means, is typically feeling very ashamed and guilty, and frequently is actively suicidal or possibly even homicidal. The first step of the caring practitioner is to provide reassurance to the patient that the practitioner will assist the patient in quietly sorting this out, and will help the patient to take the steps necessary to deal with legal and other issues. Even in the situation where the practitioner may find the behavior of the offender personally repugnant, it is inappropriate and unhelpful for the practitioner to shame the patient. At the very least, the practitioner can compliment the sex offender on sharing the information: possibly the most difficult admission a human being can make.

Sometimes an adolescent may hint that he or she has done something inappropriate or illegal. In such situations, it's helpful to remember the health practitioner's primary role is as a healer, not a lawyer, police officer or interrogator. Informing patients of their rights, limitations of confidentiality and the consequences of disclosure *prior to the disclosure* is respectful of the patient's rights and human dignity. Knowing the legal limits of confidentiality is extremely helpful here.

In situations where sex offending is suspected or even acknowledged, it is still important to get a good behavioral understanding of what has happened. Many adolescents feel guilty about all sorts of sexual experimentation, and a confession of offending or harassment should not be accepted uncritically. Key details include finding out the approximate age of the victim(s), whether the patient believed it was consensual, the actual behavior and any consequences. The practitioner may have to assist the patient to gain a realistic understanding of what happened.

Not all illegal sex acts and sex offending behaviors are reportable. For example, incest may be illegal in many jurisdictions, but some sexual exploration between same-age siblings is common. Similarly, exposing may be illegal but not reportable in many jurisdictions. Neither does all sex offending necessarily have negative impact on victims. Victim impact will vary, dependent on such factors as age of victim, victim resilience, what occurred, what degree of coercion was employed, and so forth. Hence, it's important for the practitioner not to assume that a victim has been traumatized, and also that the perpetrator was untraumatized by her or his own behavior.

During the assessment, at some point the issue arises of whether and what to tell parent(s). Frequently, this is the part the adolescent fears most. Asking the adolescent how he or she thinks the parent will react is important prior to parental disclosure. Similar to working with victims, it can be helpful when working with the adolescent perpetrator to develop a realistic plan. Options include the adolescent phoning parent(s) from the practitioner's office, the practitioner requesting the presence of the parent(s) at the office to address serious immediate concerns of the child/adolescent, and the practitioner disclosing what has happened on behalf of the adolescent.

Because many adolescents have a limited ability to realistically plan for the long term, it can be helpful in this situation to outline a usual or probable course of action. If the practitioner is unsure of what happens, she or he can ask the child protection authority, when reporting the abuse, what the adolescent can expect to happen next and then relay this to the patient (see Box 14-3).

BOX 14-3

Reassuring the minor whose behavior has been illegal

John, a 14 year old, has just disclosed that he and two other class-mates have been having younger kids (seven and eight year olds) give them blow-jobs. He came to you after one of the children said they were going to tell. While waiting for John's parents to arrive, the practitioner can summarize as follows:

'John, I'd like to review with you some of the things that are likely to happen from here on out. First, once Mum and Dad arrive, as we've agreed, you will tell them and I'll be here to support you. At some point, a police officer or child protection officer is going to want to hear your side of things. Down the road you may be charged, and you may have to go to court because what you have done is illegal. But the good news is that now you have told me what has been going on, we can work to get you the type of therapy that can help this sort of problem. I'm not an expert in this, but a person from child protection said that most boys who have molested other kids, once in treatment, do pretty well.'

Whether or not the offence is reportable, it is usually appropriate to encourage treatment for the concern, to provide referral to an appropriate psychotherapist or program specializing in adolescent sex-offending concerns, to develop a plan of action, and to assess the patient's risk to self and others. As with adults, adolescent promises to never do 'it' again are not sufficient guarantees. A clear plan must be enacted to ensure the safety of identified and potential victims.

SPECIFIC DEVELOPMENTAL CONCERNS OF CHILDHOOD AND ADOLESCENCE

Behavioral disorders

Enuresis (including bed-wetting), encopresis, separation anxiety disorder, conduct disorders, and oppositional defiant disorders are among the mental health disorders of infancy, childhood and adolescence. They are included here not because their underlying basis is sexual, but because parents

---

BOX 14-4

The effects of punishment in sexual development

The author (SR) had a client present with paraphilic cross-dressing. In taking the history, the client noted that when he was growing up, his father's preferred method of discipline was to dress the boy up as a girl complete with make-up and dress and to leave him at the local mall to walk home. As a boy of eight years, this left him feeling abandoned, confused, angry and terrified. As an adult, it was his strongest memory of this parent. At the most severe end of this continuum, such parental interventions clearly fall into the area of abuse, and the therapist has both a legal and ethical obligation to intervene (see below). But along the continuum of harmful-to-helpful interventions are many others that may fall into the grey area of unhelpful or ineffective. The role of the therapist in these cases is to encourage the parents to adopt more direct and helpful interventions. For example, if a child is anxious, instead of belittling her or him, it is more helpful to name the anxiety and provide physical reassurance. Referral of parents to parenting classes or a family therapist with specific training can also be considered.

---

historically have intervened with sexual-related interventions. When such disorders are occurring, it is always helpful to ask during a basic assessment how the parents usually handle the concern, how they handle it when they are at the maximum breaking point, and how they discipline their child. Whether using positive expectations, 'Jose, you need to be a man, now, because Mummy and Daddy are leaving' or punishment, 'Mary, if you're going to wet your bed like a baby, we're going to treat you as a baby', parents should be educated about the effects of their interventions. A basic rule of parenting children is never to belittle the child. Box 14-4 provides a case study of the effects of punishment on sexual development.

Body and genital image

Another common concern in puberty and adolescence regards body and genital image. Issues may range from mild discomfort and self-conscious-

---

BOX 14-5

Screening questions for body and genital image concerns for a medical practitioner

1. How do you feel about your body and the changes that are occurring?
2. (During a genital exam) Your penis/testicles/vagina look just fine—healthy and normal. Because so many men/women have concerns about how their genitals look, I usually take this opportunity to ask if you have any specific questions or concerns.
3. What do you like most about your body? What do you like least? Is there anything you would want to change if you could?

---

ness about body changes to severe problems including anorexia, bulimia and genital mutilation. Teenage girls are at the highest risk for development of eating disorders, followed by gay males. Other body image concerns include the use of steroids to body build. Screening questions for body image concerns appear in Box 14-5. Practitioners suspecting eating disorders should consider the literature linking sexual abuse as a common antecedent, take a relevant history, and refer to a specialist as appropriate.

Paraphilic development and expression

Sexual discovery is part of the normal developmental tasks of puberty and adolescence. While for most children, particularly boys, this involves the development of normophilic behaviors including masturbation, discovery of pornography, same-sex sexual experimentation and other sexual experimentation, for some children it is also a time of paraphilic experimentation and onset of paraphilias. By definition, 'paraphilia' is the term used to describe behaviors beyond the norm, ranging from the uncommon to the bizarre. These include those listed in the DSM-IV (e.g., exposing, voyeuring, fetishes, obscene phone calling, toucherism, sexual contact with much younger children, and frotteurism) as well as more unconventional expressions (storing of urine in jars, uncommon fetishes, binding of genitalia, rape and sadistic urges, and autoerotic asphyxia).

In treating the adolescent with paraphilic behavior, it is important to remember several things. First, it is never appropriate to criticize, blame or laugh at an adolescent's sexual health concerns. Belittling or shaming the adolescent increases the risk of suicide attempts as well as further eroticizing the paraphilia. Rather, a reassuring, open, non-judgmental approach is recommended. Second, by definition the compulsive aspects to the behavior are unlikely to cease simply because you or a parent tells the adolescent not to do it. This just drives the behavior 'underground'. It is more helpful to thank the adolescent for disclosing what is happening, and to express your willingness to help the adolescent understand himself or herself and why this behavior is so powerful and/or erotic to him or her.

Third, it can be helpful to remember that compulsive sexual behaviors typically provide an anxiety-reduction and/or self-punishment function. While many paraphilias become eroticized, it is not accurate to assume that the patient experiences the behavior as erotic. Similarly, normophilic behaviors can become compulsively driven. Some adolescents experience negative effects because of their sexual behavior; for example, being seen by peers as sexually promiscuous, socially ostracized or in legal trouble because of sexually inappropriate comments or behavior. In such cases, the practitioner should treat the case with appropriate concern, assess the problem and the adolescent's rationale for why it is occurring, and consider referral to an adolescent sexual health specialist as appropriate.

Fourth, it is important to get an accurate sexual history of what else is going on. It is useful to remember that non-contact offending behaviors—exhibitionism, voyeurism, obscene phone calls, other sexual harassment—are highly intercorrelated. In taking the history, focus first on the presenting behavior (when it started, why the patient thinks it started, how it developed, how frequently it happens, and what are the important, powerful and/or disturbing characteristics of this behavior to the patient) and then focus on other behaviors, asking about specific examples if necessary.

Fifth, it is important to ask specific questions about any other behaviors that may be damaging or harmful to the patient or others. Where there is threat of imminent harm—a patient who may be mutilating or harming his or her genitals or a patient admitting autoerotic asphyxia, for example—immediate professional assessment and hospitalization may be required. In other cases, where there is a serious negative impact or impact potential for the patient, referral to a specialist is recommended.

Treatment typically includes pharmacotherapy (to decrease the compulsive elements), psychotherapy (to assist the patient to identify what factors and co-factors maintain the paraphilia, as well as to identify an alternate satisfying plan for sexual activity), and social support. Where specialist treatment is not available, treating under the consultation of a specialist should be considered the alternative standard of care. Treatment should have dual goals: to treat the paraphilia, and to promote normophilic development.

Two mistakes are common. The first is to jump to conclusions and assume something is paraphilic when it is not. It saves a lot of time and wasted energy to ask the adolescents if they know why they are engaging in this behavior (see Box 14-6). A second mistake is to minimize the seriousness of certain behaviors, especially exhibitionism and voyeurism. While many adolescents may act out by occasionally 'mooning', 'streaking' or 'peeking', the adolescent with a pattern of exposing or voyeurism is engaging in a behavior that has negative legal and social consequences. It is very important that the patient receive a consistent message about what behaviors are acceptable and what behaviors are problematic. Paraphilic behaviors are extremely difficult to treat successfully. Some researchers believe the societal mixed messages regarding exhibitionism and voyeurism explain, at

---

BOX 14-6
When is a paraphilia not a paraphilia?

A developmentally delayed adolescent in supervised care was referred for suspected copraphilic tendencies. He had been observed masturbating repeatedly using his feces as lubricant. Because this led to the patient smelling of feces post-masturbation, the behavior had negative social as well as potential health impact. Staff decided to consult a psychologist specializing in sex, and his case worker was advised to quietly ask the adolescent why he engaged in this activity.

The adolescent was not able to provide much help, beyond saying it felt good. Eventually, the case worker asked him why he didn't use spit (like most adolescent boys). The adolescent became quite indignant, informing the case worker that he had been taught he wasn't allowed to spit.

In this case, what looked like a paraphilia was an adolescent trying to obey rules while achieving some sexual pleasuring. Staff providing the adolescent with lubricant was all that was needed to treat the presenting concern.

least in part, why these behaviors have one of the poorest prognoses of any paraphilia for successful treatment.

HEALTH CARE FOR THE DEVELOPING LESBIAN, GAY, BISEXUAL AND TRANSGENDERED CHILD AND ADOLESCENT

It must be noted with regret that in the past many health interventions for developing lesbian, gay, bisexual and transgendered children and adolescents were useless at best, and harmful at worst. The common mistakes of practitioners were denial ('No, I don't think this means you're X'), minimization ('You're not really gay/lesbian/bisexual/transgender; this is just a stage you're going through'), pathologization ('I'm very worried about you. Do you want to get AIDS?'), avoidance ('Well, I'm not the right one to talk to about that') and betrayal ('I'm going to talk with your parents about what you have just told me'). All are inappropriate and potentially harmful to patients. To a greater or lesser extent, what these interventions do is to take the patient's reality, filter it through a highly trusted and credible source (the health practitioner), and send back to the patient a confusing, distorting picture. The next two sections focus on how to counsel in situations where same-sex behavior is the presenting concern.

Adolescent homosexual behavior

The first step for practitioners is to develop a realistic understanding of the tasks of adolescence and the normality of same-sex and other-sex exploration.

Across countries and cultures, some same-sex sexual experience in adolescence appears common. The 1988 American National Survey of Adolescent Males, drawing on a representative sample of non-institutionalized, never-married males between 15 and 19 years, reported that 3% 'had engaged in homosexual activity'.[18] Sorenson[19] found 17% of boys and 6% of girls between 16 and 19 years reported at least one homosexual experience. These figures should not be taken as representative of adolescents with sexual orientation concerns, as many adolescents cope with same-sex feelings and desires by avoiding any behavior, especially homosexual sexual behavior, that would confirm their sexual orientation.

Where adolescents have less access to sexual experimentation with the other gender—for example, in single-sex boarding schools, clubs and social networks—the incidence of same-sex experimentation is thought to be much higher. (It's not that single-sex boarding schools or the boy scouts 'create' homosexuality; adolescence is a powerfully sexual time, and many adolescents and youths seek outlets for their sexual drive. It appears that people are sexual beings, first. If one only has access to one or other gender, then one modifies one's behavior accordingly.) The meaning of same-sex behavior may also vary by sexual orientation. Retrospective studies of adults suggest that while for many heterosexually identified adults some homosexual activity in adolescence is forgotten, remembered as an outlet for frustrated sexual expression, or remembered fondly as fun and relief, for many homosexually identified adults their early homosexual experiences coincided with falling in love, confronting their sexual orientation, beginning the 'coming out' process, or being 'outed'. Hence, when an adolescent reveals some homosexual behavior, or parents reveal their knowledge of it, it is important to not assume, based on the behavior alone, the sexual orientation of the patient. It's also important when an adolescent raises homosexual behavior issues to consider these issues as important and not to dismiss them outright as a passing phase. Asking adolescents what the behavior means for them, helping them to gently explore the implications of their behavior, and when necessary providing multiple interpretations of the behavior, will be more helpful. 'Well, from what you've told me, it may mean that you're attracted to men/women, or this may be something that changes as you develop. What would it mean for you if it turns out you are attracted to other boys/girls?'

Adolescent sexual orientation

One of the most important tasks of adolescence is to develop an accurate self-awareness of one's sexuality. The practitioner's role is two-fold: first, to be aware of normal developmental tasks and affirm these (see chapter 13); and second, to be aware of risk factors and co-factors for adolescent sexual minorities.

Few studies have been able to assess the prevalence of various sexual orientations in adolescents. A Minnesota study of 34 706 students aged 13–18 years, using representative sampling methods, found that 88% defined themselves as predominantly heterosexual, 11% as unsure, and 1% as bisexual or predominantly homosexual.[20] Based on this study, the alert practitioner should assume that for at least one in ten adolescents, sexual orientation concerns are relevant.

Recent research has begun to assess the impact of youths' sexual identity on suicide risk. In a study of 137 gay and bisexual adolescents, 41 (30%) reported a suicide attempt, and almost half of these reported multiple attempts.[21] According to the authors, over half the attempts were moderate to severe (in terms of lethality). However, only 21% of attempts resulted in medical or psychiatric admissions. Adolescents at increased risk were males with more feminine gender roles, and those who had adopted a homosexual or bisexual identity at a younger age. Attempters were more likely to report sexual abuse, drug abuse and arrests for misconduct. Remafedi and colleagues[21] note that one third of the suicide attempts were attributed to personal or interpersonal turmoil about homosexuality, and one third of first attempts occurred in the same year that subjects identified their bisexuality or homosexuality. Clearly, the earliest stages of coming out (Coleman's[22] pre-coming-out stage and coming-out stage) should be considered a period of high suicide risk for minors. In particular, adolescents who come out in early and middle teenage years may be less able to cope with the isolation and stigma of a homosexual identity, and family problems were the most frequently cited reason for attempts.

One in three suicide attempts in childhood and adolescence are thought to be related to sexual orientation concerns, yet sexual orientation itself is not a risk factor.[21] Rather, abuse experienced because of one's perceived sexual orientation, disturbed family dynamics, rejection by significant others and internalized homophobia are considered the major risk factors. It is important, first, to assess each of these factors, and second, to intervene if necessary. In the home, school and other situations, it's important to assess whether the patient feels safe (physically and sexually), and respected, as these will predict the suicide risk. This also sends an affirming message to the patient that the health practitioner is not just concerned about a patient's diseases, but is concerned about all matters related to health.

It's important not to dismiss socially common events as unimportant. The child or adolescent who routinely experiences the playground as a place where she or he is called 'faggot' and is beaten, is not uncommon; every school may have one or several children who is bullied and abused on a daily basis. The health practitioner has an important role as patient advocate here. With the adolescent's permission, the practitioner can encourage the parents, or the adolescent if necessary, to intervene. Even without the patient's permission, in situations of significant harm, the practitioner may still be required to disclose the danger while protecting the patient's identity. In practice, this sometimes comes down to a balancing of the patient's right to privacy and the practitioner's duty to disclose in situations of harm. A helpful principle is 'need to know': that even in a situation of danger, the therapist should think about how much information others—parents, school, other authorities—need to know. For example, in a situation where an adolescent cross-dresser is being bullied and/or raped, it may not be necessary to mention the adolescent's cross-dressing.

Sometimes the health professional may be approached on matters tangential, but not unrelated, to sexual orientation. Many adolescents dread sports and changing-room activities required in many school curricula. Body and genital image concerns and intimidation are common, regardless of sexual orientation. For the patient questioning her or his sexual orientation or emerging as gay or lesbian, additional terrors exist. For males in particular, fear of getting an erection while having to change and shower may precipitate avoidant behaviors. Part of psychological and mental health is feeling safe. The adolescent who fears being outed—including by his own physical response—should have that fear respected. If necessary, the health practitioner should write a note excusing the patient from such activities. As well, the practitioner can work with the adolescent on alternative ways the adolescent can socialize and achieve physical exercise goals.

The counselling of adolescents regarding sexual orientation concerns mirrors that discussed in the previous chapter on the sexual orientation concerns of adults, but there are other ways in which the practitioner can be helpful. Several novels for adolescents that include gay and lesbian characters have now been published. Practitioners can recommend age-appropriate reading which in turn provides role modelling and positive expectations for the patient. Encouraging the adolescent to see you on a regular basis 'even if you don't have anything wrong with you' is also appropriate. These adolescents have been identified as being at higher risk, and hence preventive health interventions are appropriate. Informing the adolescent about gay/lesbian support groups and other health care services is helpful. Although some practitioners fear this may precipitate sexual activity, for adolescents at high risk, contact with similar others is essential to prevent isolation and further suicide attempts. For practitioners who may not specialize in seeing adolescents, counselling of children and adolescents generally needs to proceed at a slower pace than counselling with adults. Confidentiality concerns of adolescents are frequently much greater. It's important that the practitioner respects the confidentiality concerns of the adolescent, and explains the limits of confidentiality with the patient. Helping the adolescent to deal with pressure to be sexual, respecting his or her stage of psychosexual development, and encouraging the adolescent to develop positive self-esteem and identity in other areas, are all important. Decisions to delay experimentation should be respected. For example, the adolescent who decides not to explore his or her sexuality at that time because of the need to study hard to get into medical or law school should have these decisions affirmed.

In most cases, the psychosexual development of the lesbian or gay identified adolescent will occur at the same stage as—or at an earlier stage than—that of their heterosexual counterparts. Hence, the practitioner can use the same questions she or he would use for heterosexually identified adolescents. In addition, in the early stages of coming out, it is sometimes helpful to affirm the adolescent's self-disclosure by using gender-specific terms. For example, 'Peter, given that you've been exploring your attractions to other males, let's talk about what kind of guys you really like, and what your ideal man for the future might be'. Because lesbian or gay adolescents have usually not had the opportunity to discuss openly their dreams, ideals and desires, the health professional may need to create opportunities for them to catch up with their peer group.

In summary, childhood and adolescence are times of sexual discovery, exploration and development. Yet, historically, counselling by health practitioners has been ineffective and even harmful. The health practitioner has multiple roles involving the sexual counselling of children and adolescents. For most patients, assisting the minor patient and parents to integrate sexual health into their physical, mental, emotional and other aspects of health is important. The practitioner may need to develop additional skills to appropriately and effectively address the sexual concerns of minors. Some situations such as abuse are complex ethically and legally, and the health professional is advised to seek assistance and expert referral in such situations. Other situations identify children and adolescents at higher risk of suicide; here the practitioner can play an important and helpful role as patient advocate, and in assisting the minor and his or her family to deal with the minor's sexual concerns.

REFERENCES

1. U.S. National Institutes of Health. *NIH consensus statement on interventions to prevent HIV risk behaviors.* Bethesda, MD: U.S, Government, 1997: 1–20.
2. Povinelli, M., Remafedi, G. and Tao, G. Trends and predictors of human immunodeficiency virus antibody testing by homosexual and bisexual adolescent males, 1989–1994. *Archives of Pediatric Medicine*, 1996; 150: 33–38.
3. Rawitscher, L.E., Saitz, R. and Friedman, L.S. Adolescents' preferences regarding human immunodeficiency virus (HIV)-related practitioner counseling and HIV testing. *Pediatrics*, 1995; 96: 52–57.
4. Hingson, R., Strunin, L. and Berlin, B. Acquired immunodeficiency syndrome transmission: Changes in knowledge and behaviors among teenagers. Massachusetts statewide surveys, 1986–1988. *Pediatrics*, 1990; 85: 24–29.
5. Shuster, M.A., Bell, R.M., Petersen, L.P. and Kanouse, D.E. Communication between adolescents and physicians about sexual risk behavior. *Archives of Pediatric and Adolescent Medicine*, 1996; 150: 906–913.
6. Calabrese, L.H., Kelley, D.M., Collen, R.J. and Locker, G. Physician's atti-

tudes, beliefs, and practices regarding health care promotion. *Archives of Internal Medicine*, 1991; 151: 1157–1160.

7. Fredman, L., Rabic, D., Bowman, M., Bandermer, C., Sardeson, K., Taggart, V.S. and English, D.K. Primary care physicians: assessment and prevention of HIV infection. *American Journal of Preventive Medicine*, 1989; 5: 188–195.

8. Society for Adolescent Medicine. Access to health care for adolescents: a position paper of the Society for Adolescent Medicine. *Journal of Adolescent Health*, 1998; 13: 162–170.

9. U.S. Public Health Service. *Healthy People 2000*. Hyattsville, MD: U.S. Department of Health and Human Services, Public Health Service, 1991.

10. U.S. Preventive Services Task Force. Guide to clinical preventive services: an assessment of the effectiveness of 169 interventions. *Report of the U.S. Preventive Services Task Force*. Baltimore: Williams & Wilkins, 1989.

11. American Medical Association. *Information report of the council of scientific affairs*. Chicago: American Medical Association, 1988.

12. American Medical Association. Oral and written submission to the *NIH Consensus Development Conference on Interventions to Prevent HIV Risk Behaviors*. Bethesda, MD: National Institutes of Health, 1997.

13. American College of Physicians and Infectious Diseases Society of America. Human immunodeficiency virus (HIV) infection. *Annals of Internal Medicine*, 1994; 120: 310–319.

14. American Academy of Family Physicians. *1993–1994 compendium of AAFP positions on selected health issues*. Kansas City, Mo: American Academy of Family Physicians, 1993.

15. American College of Obstetricians and Gynecologists. The adolescent obstetrician-gynecologic patients. *American College of Obstetricians and Gynecologists Technical Bulletin*, 1986; 84: 1–5.

16. Elster, A.B. and Kuzsets, N. Guidelines for adolescent preventive services (GAPS). Baltimore, MD: Williams and Wilkins, 1993.

17. Finkelhor, D., Hotaling, Lewis, and Smith. Sexual abuse in a national survey of adult men and women. *Child Abuse and Neglect*, 1990: 14: 19–28.

18. Sonenstein, F.L., Pleck, J.H. and Ku, I.C. Sexual activity, condom use, and AIDS awareness among adolescent males. *Family Planning Perspectives*, 1989; 21: 152–158.

19. Sorenson, R.C. *Adolescent Sexuality in Contemporary America*. New York, NY: World Publishing, 1973: 285–295.

20. Remafedi, G., Resnick, M., Blum, R. and Harris, L. Demography of sexual orientation in adolescents. *Pediatrics*, 1992; 90: 714–721.

21. Remafedi, G., Farrow, J.A. and Deisher, R.W. Risk factors for attempted suicide in gay and bisexual youth. *Pediatrics*, 1991; 87: 869–875.

22. Coleman, E. Development stages of the coming-out process. *American Behavioral Scientist*, 1974; 25: 469–482.

15 *Sexuality and aging*

Perhaps the most positive attitude to aging and sex is that taken by Loulan,[1] who maintains that, over the years, people learn from experience how to pleasure partners and what they themselves find pleasing. Sex can only get better. Nevertheless, aging is undoubtedly accompanied by physical and physiological effects, and some of these can affect sexuality in a negative way. For males, the gradual reduction in testosterone production can reduce libido, slow sexual responses and perhaps be implicated in erectile dysfunction. For women, the impact of menopause can be more dramatic, occurring as it does in a shorter time frame. It is worth remarking, though, that relatively few women suffer libido loss or vaginal symptoms that make intercourse difficult or painful.

Perhaps the two most significant factors that affect sexuality are partner availability and the individual's image as a person and a sexual being. The most common reason given by post-menopausal women for discontinuing intercourse is loss of a partner through death or separation.[2] This is likely to be true for men as well. Given the shorter life-span of the human male, women are more likely to find themselves bereaved and more likely to have difficulty in finding another male partner. Perhaps even more important in discontinuation of sexual relations is the fact that older people may view themselves as being unattractive and non-sexual beings. This is not at all an unrealistic perception in general social terms (see Box 15-1). Still, as discussed throughout this book, it's important for practitioners to realize that people are individuals and that their responses to physical, psychological and psychosocial changes vary enormously. Be prepared to question in a matter-of-fact way and to listen carefully to the answers you receive.

FACTORS TO CONSIDER IN COUNSELLING THE OLDER PATIENT

Factors in the partnership

A major psychosocial change experienced by older people is the retirement of one or both partners. The psychological impact of retirement may be a

---

BOX 15-1

The sexual image of older people

A friend is a divorced woman of 70. During a routine visit to her medical practitioner, she requested an HIV test. 'But, why?' asked the practitioner, in total astonishment. She claims to have resisted the temptation to say, 'Why do you think, Sonny?'.

---

feeling that one is no longer useful, no longer powerful. And, of course, people may find themselves with much less disposable income. In addition, couples will have a lot more time to spend with each other. For some people, activities previously regarded as hobbies may move to a central position in their life. For many people, however, the initial adjustment period may evolve into a major problem in filling increased time at home. A partner who has already retired or who has never worked may resent changes to routine and increased demands in terms of personal interactive time, food preparation and so on.

Retired people have a widening opportunity as regards the times when they can have sex. On the other hand, one or both partners may experience decreasing libido or simple boredom with an oft-repeated scenario; these and other factors may be reflected in a decrease in intercourse frequency. The important question here is whether or not the changes occur in parallel in both partners. It should be noted that 55.8% of a sample of post-menopausal women rated an active sex life as 'important'.[2] The figures for men are not available, but one would hardly expect them to be lower.

Chronic illness or injury

Sexual intercourse can be uncomfortable or painful for patients experiencing chronic pain or injury (see chapter 9). With increasing age, people are more likely to develop long-term degenerative diseases such as arthritis and rheumatism, and to suffer from the long-term effects of injuries previously incurred in sporting activities and motor vehicle accidents. The side effects of medication may depress libido or cause tiredness. One partner may be afraid of hurting the other. And the illness may be used to avoid sex, if that is what the sufferer wants. Several modifications can be made so that people can ensure they are able to continue an active sex life. As so often happens, clients may be reluctant to raise the sexual implications of illness sponta-

---

BOX 15-2

Sexual advice for patients with chronic illness or pain

- Make sure that you time sex to happen when your pain medication is at its most effective.
- Have sex at the time of day when it suits you, when you are likely to feel your best.
- Be ready to tell your partner when something hurts, in a calm way. Move on to some more relaxing sexual activity rather than shutting down abruptly.
- Experiment with different positions for intercourse. Use lots of pillows to support you in a comfortable position.
- Try manual or oral sex.
- Consider pleasuring just one partner.

Derived from: *Living and Loving: Information about Sex.* Arthritis Foundation of USA, 1990.

---

neously. This is especially true when someone suspects that his or her partner is using the illness as a sexual 'out'. The role of the health practitioner is, as ever, to bring the topic into the consultation in a calm, professional manner and to be prepared for clients who simply prefer to keep this part of their lives private. Advice on sexual functioning for patients experiencing chronic pain or injury is detailed in Box 15-2.

Recovery from stroke and heart attack

Sexual activity causes a rather dramatic rise in blood pressure. It is not surprising then that many strokes and heart attacks occur during sexual intercourse. People may well believe that resuming their physical sex life after a stroke or heart attack may be dangerous. As a rule of thumb, Goble[3] suggests that after heart attack, if a male client can walk a kilometre (half a mile or so) comfortably or climb two flights of stairs without getting breathless, then sexual activity should be safe for him. He puts this in a time frame of about three weeks. Goble also suggests that clients resume the same patterns of sexual intercourse in terms of timing, frequency and position. As ever, individual variation is important here. It depends very much on the degree of physical exertion that sexual activity entails.

Sexual Health Concerns: Interviewing and History Taking

BOX 15-3

Questions to ask after heart attack or stroke

- Tell me about your sexual activity before this happened. (Probes: Partner(s)? Frequency? Enjoyment and satisfaction?)
- What did the doctor who treated you tell you about sexual activity afterwards? (Probes: Physical signs of readiness to resume sex? Time frame? Chances of recurrence? Medication effects?)
- Have you resumed sexual activity? (Probes: What did you do? How did it go? Any anxieties for you? Anxieties for your partner?)
- How are you feeling? (Probes: Tiredness? Anxiety? Depression?)
- How has this affected your lifestyle? (Probes: Changes in physical activity? Changes in household task allocation? Changes in decision making? Financial implications?)

Another central change after stroke / heart attack may occur in the power structure of the relationship. The sufferer may be pushed into the sick role and perceive a loss of power on many fronts. The partner may feel resentful about increased physical and emotional demands. It is essential to ask about reallocation of responsibilities and tasks and their effects on both partners. Box 15-3 lists questions to ask after heart attack or stroke.

Bereavement and separation

As with retirement, bereavement or separation entails a major period of adjustment. Especially for heterosexual women, finding a new partner may be difficult. For many people, it is an option they simply do not want to consider. (A client kindly gave LDC-L a tip on husband-hunting should her marriage break up. 'Go to a meeting of Alcoholics Anonymous in a posh suburb. Their marriages busted up while they were on the booze and they're all looking for understanding women.' I'm not sure to what extent we should pass on this advice.) The practitioner's role is to give permission to discuss sexuality, while treading the fine line of not invading privacy (see Box 15-4). Masturbation may be an important subject here, and should be introduced in a matter-of-fact way. For many clients, it may be a distaste-

---

BOX 15-4

Questions to ask in bereavement or separation

- How are you coping with day-to-day life? (Probes: New tasks? Financial? Other family members?)
- How are you feeling? (Probes: Loneliness? Anxiety? Depression? Anger?)
- Have their been any changes in your social life? (Probes: Old friends? New friends? Activities?)
- What is happening in your sex life? (Probes: Efforts to find new partner? Skills in initiating a new relationship? Self-image? Masturbation?)

---

ful topic, or one that during grieving may seem to violate the memory of their partner. However, some women are cheered by the information that, in the absence of a partner, masturbation is a healthy activity which maintains the elasticity of the vaginal mucosa.

Sleeping arrangements

Many couples prefer to sleep in separate bedrooms or separate beds at this stage of life. Pain from illness or injury may make for restless sleep, which can disturb a partner. Snoring and sleep apnea increase with age in males and post-menopausally in females. Separate beds can make sex more of an occasion, which can have positive or negative results. Once again, open communication between partners is essential.

ISSUES IN AGING FOR WOMEN

The mean age of menopause in western society is 51.5 years. Dramatic though menopause may be, most women are well aware of the effects of aging before that. A friend described a woman's forties as 'a cruel decade'. Facial and bodily wrinkles increase; there is a tendency to put on weight. If you elect to stay slim, you tend to look facially haggard. As Germaine Greer[4] put it in her inimitable way, 'It's your face or your bum'.

In contrast to the gradual changes occurring in male endocrine levels as a man ages, the relatively rapid involution of the ovaries and decrease in oestrogen levels produce some notable changes in a relatively short space of time. Perhaps the most distressing symptom is hot flashes, a sudden increase in body temperature with attendant sweating, flushing and possibly chilling afterwards. Some women find they become emotionally labile at this time. Small incidents that they would previously have taken in their stride can reduce them to tears. Other women find they become vague and forgetful. A colleague who specializes in menopause describes this as 'the handbag in the fridge syndrome'. All of this can be exacerbated by concurrent stress. Difficulties with aging and ill parents, job problems, her retirement or the retirement of her partner, and children's life problems can simply make things worse.

Vaginal and sexual problems

About 10% of women of menopausal age or older suffer vaginal atrophy, which can result in painful intercourse. Some women avoid sexual intercourse because of this, and the partner may feel rejected and sexually frustrated. Another cause of painful intercourse at this time of life is vaginal dryness: it may simply take longer for the woman to become sexually aroused and lubricated. Sometimes there is little lubrication in spite of arousal. Water-based lubricants, available in supermarkets and pharmacies, are often effective, if somewhat unromantic and messy. A high proportion of women presenting at menopause clinics show loss of libido,[2] and this can have disruptive effects on the relationship. However, for other women the removal of the risk of pregnancy has the positive effect of allowing them to relax and enjoy intercourse more. Whenever you encounter loss of libido in a patient, be alert for the possibility of depression as a contributing factor. Box 15-5 suggests some questions to ask older women.

Hormone replacement therapy

For women, the question arises whether or not to take hormone replacement therapy. Oestrogen replacement is likely to reduce hot flashes, give a woman control of irregular menstruation and iron out some of the emotionality. It may help reduce vaginal dryness and soreness and increase lubrication in sexual arousal. In the early days of hormone replacement therapy, an increase in endometrial cancer was found in women using it. This occurred at a time when oestrogen alone was prescribed. More recently, oestrogen accompanied by a progesterone has largely been the therapy of

BOX 15-5

Questions to ask older women

- Has the frequency with which you have had intercourse changed over the past few years? Can you think of any reasons for this? (Probes: Libido loss? Partner's libido loss? Loss of partner? Sleeping arrangement changes?)
- Has your enjoyment of sexual intercourse changed since your menopause? (Probes: Increased? Decreased? How does your partner feel about this?)
- Have you experienced painful intercourse of late? (Probes: Arousal level? Lubrication?)
- Have you noticed any changes in the way your partner behaves during sexual intercourse? (Probes: General affection and enthusiasm? Erectile problems?)
- Is there anything stressful in your life at the moment? (Probes: Job? Partner's job? Finances? Parents' health, relationships, living arrangements, finances? Children's health, relationships, jobs, finances?)
- When was your last mammogram? When was your last Pap smear? (Probes: Discomfort? Embarrassment?)

choice. In this situation, no increased risk or a very slight increase in incidence is seen.[5] The relationship between breast cancer incidence and hormone replacement therapy remains equivocal. For many women, the enhanced quality of day-to-day life is worth any slight increase in risk.

Some feminist writers, notably Germaine Greer,[4] argue firmly that the use of hormone replacement therapy imposes unnecessary disease status on menopause. Greer proposes that hormone replacement therapy prevents women from making a smooth transition to older age by artificially putting back the hormonal clock. As far as cardiovascular risk is concerned, hormone replacement therapy may actually prevent or arrest its development, particularly in the case of atherosclerosis.[5,6]

Hormone replacement therapy can reduce calcium loss—and the subsequent loss of bone density that puts a woman at increased risk of hip and leg fractures as she ages—but only in the context of regular weight-bearing exercise and a diet that is rich in calcium.

Breast and uterine cancer

For both these cancers, early detection is related to lower mortality. Especially if a woman has a family history of breast cancer, monthly self-examination of the breasts and annual mammograms are necessary. Australian health authorities recommend annual mammograms for all women over 50. Pap smears at one- or two-year intervals for the early detection of uterine cancer are similarly suggested. Many women find that both of these investigations constitute something of an invasion of privacy. They can also be uncomfortable if not downright painful. Prior to conducting examinations physicians should ask about previous tests and any history of patient discomfort or pain. While some minimal physical discomfort during a mammogram is common, a Pap smear ought not to be painful. Where patients report a history of discomfort or pain, the physician can then take extra care to redress the patient's experience.

ISSUES IN AGING FOR MEN

While the emphasis on youthful good looks is usually less for men than for women in western society, it is nonetheless an issue. The gradual waning of physical strength is also a reminder of the passage of time. Men tend to compare their current level of physical strength with that of their youth and find it irritatingly reduced: 'I can't lift a bag of concrete any more'. Obesity can also become a problem, with a majority of western men putting on weight from their early forties. The desirability of maintaining a healthy non-fluctuating weight, however, seems to have had little impact on the dietary habits of middle-aged men. Stress adds to any other problems. For some retired men, boredom is a highly potent stressor. Financial problems, failing health, problems with partner or children, can all interact.

Sexual functioning

The gradual reduction in testosterone production has less impact in the male than the rapid involution of the ovaries has in women, but still affects physical and sexual function. (Some have suggested that testosterone replacement therapy may be useful, but adequate research on its value is not yet published.) Older men may take longer to become physically aroused and develop an erection sufficient to have sexual intercourse. They may take longer to ejaculate and may produce less volume of semen than in their earlier years. In addition, they may not feel the need to ejaculate every time they have sexual intercourse. For many partners, this makes sex a more relaxed and unhurried experience, especially if the man is not troubled with performance anxiety.

Some men notice changes in the appearance of their erect penis as they age, commonly a bend to one side or the other. Peyronie's disease, as it is known, is the result of the growth of fibrous tissue along the shaft of the penis, possibly caused by minor injury to the penis during intercourse. If it causes pain on erection or makes intercourse difficult, a consultation with a urologist is called for.

Erectile difficulties

Some men may experience difficulties getting or maintaining an erection sufficient for intercourse. It is useful to check whether they experience any erections at all, for example nocturnal ones. If they do, it is likely that psychological factors such as performance anxiety or boredom with routine sexual activities may be involved. Many older men are taking medications that also affect erections, so it is important to determine what drugs the man is taking (see Box 15-6).

Prostate disease

About half the population of men over 50 will show some enlargement of the prostate gland. Usually this is benign and, unless it causes problems such as frequent urination or difficulty urinating, most authorities recommend that it be left alone. Apart from skin cancer, prostate cancer is the

---

BOX 15-6
A quick fix for erectile dysfunction

Asked what prescribed medications he was taking, a client who presented to a psychotherapist with erectile dysfunction listed what sounded like a formula for disaster: antihypertensives, diuretics and tranquillizers. 'Could you outline the problem to your medical practitioner and ask advice about the effects of your medication?' I asked. 'But I can't talk to him about that—he's our family doctor.' He did, however, pluck up courage to ask and rang to cancel his next appointment. A reduction in the diuretic medication had had an immediate impact on his erectile functioning.

BOX 15-7

Questions to ask older men

- Has the frequency with which you have had intercourse changed over the past few years? Can you think of any reasons for this? (Probes: Libido loss? Erectile difficulties? Partner's libido loss? Loss of partner? Sleeping arrangement changes?)
- Has your enjoyment of sexual intercourse changed over the past few years? (Probes: Increased? Decreased? How does your partner feel about this?)
- Have you experienced painful intercourse of late? (Probes: Peyronie-type changes to the penis? Partner's lubrication?)
- Have you noticed any changes in the way your partner behaves during sexual intercourse? (Probes: Enthusiasm? Lubrication? Orgasm?)
- Have you noticed any changes in your erect penis? (Probes: Degree of hardness? Bending?)
- Do you have any difficulty with urination? (Probes: Frequency? Quality of stream? Nocturnal waking?)
- Have you ever been examined for prostate cancer? (Probes: Physical examination? PSA test? Findings?)
- Have there been any major changes to your lifestyle over the past few years? (Probes: Partner disharmony? Retirement? Moving house? Children's troubles?) Have you found any of these changes stressful?

---

most frequently reported carcinoma in older men. A blood test (Prostate Specific Antigen test or PSA) is now available for the diagnosis and monitoring of prostate disease. Since the test became available in the 1980s, the incidence of reported prostate cancer has increased. Prostate mortality, however, remains unchanged.[7] Unlike the case with breast and uterine cancer, early detection does not seem to be linked to greater treatment success. Because of this, the recommendation in Australia is that it not be used as a routine screening test in older men[8] to avoid exposing them to unnecessary anxiety and unhelpful intervention.

Prostate surgery for benign or cancerous enlargement commonly results in retrograde ejaculation. Semen travels backwards into the bladder at ejaculation rather than out of the penis. Men who experience this mainly report that their experience of climax is unchanged or perhaps only slightly diminished in spite of the dry orgasm. Surgery may also be associated with urinary incontinence. It is worthwhile to inform men and their partners about these likely changes pre-operatively and to be prepared to discuss them after recovery from surgery. A personalised and informative review of prostate problems is given in Llewellyn-Jones.[9] Questions to ask the older man are reviewed in Box 15-7.

REFERENCES

1. Lulan, J. *Lesbian Sex*. San Francisco: spinsters/aunt lute, 1984.
2. Channon, L.D and Ballinger, S.E. Some aspects of sexuality and vaginal symptoms during menopause and their relation to anxiety and depression. *British Journal of Medical Psychology*, 1986; 59: 173–180.
3. Goble, A. Sexual function after myocardial infarction. *Current Therapeutics*, 1997; 38: 73–75.
4. Greer, G. *The Change. Women, Ageing and the Menopause*. London: Hamish Hamilton, 1991.
5. Weiss, N.S and Hill, D.A. Postmenopausal estrogens and progestogens and the incidence of gynaecological cancer. *Maturitas*, 1996; 23: 235–239.
6. Punnonen, R.H., Jokela, H.A., Dastidar, P.S., Nevela, M. and Laipalla, P.J. Combined oestrogen-progestin replacement therapy prevents atherosclerosis in postmenopausal women. *Maturitas*, 1995; 21: 179–187.
7. Smith, D.P. and Armstrong, B.K. Prostate-specific antigen testing in Australia and association with prostate cancer incidence in New South Wales. *Medical Journal of Australia*, 1998; 169: 17–20.
8. Kramer, B.S., Gohagan, J.K. and Prorok, P.C. Is screening for prostate cancer the current gold standard?—'No.'. *European Journal of Cancer*, 1997; 33: 348–353.
9. Llewellyn-Jones, D. *Your prostate. An owner's manual*. Ringwood, Vic.: Penguin, Australia 1997.

Index

abortion, 25–6
abstinence, 188–9, 190
active listening, 53, 54–5
adolescents
  behavioral disorders, 194–5, 196–9
  body image, 195–6, 202
  homosexuality, 199–203
  legal considerations in treating, 8, 158, 190,
    191, 192
  paraphilias, 196–9
  parental disclosure, 193
  practitioner–patient language, 23, 182, 187
  sex education, 188
  sexual abuse, 190–4
  sexual counselling, 182–203
  and sexual history taking, 8, 15, 23, 24,
    182–4, 197
  as sexual offenders, 192–4
  sexual orientation concerns, 200–3
  and STDs, 188–9
  suicide, 200–2, 203
alcohol
  effects on sexual function, 65, 122, 126–7
  and risk behaviors, 118–19
  see also drugs
anal intercourse and STDs, 45, 46, 134, 173
anorgasmia, 27, 28–9, 35, 36, 75–80
autoimmune disease (AIDS) see HIV/AIDS

behavioral counselling
  definition, 51–2
  interventions in sexual dysfunction, 60–72,
    73–81
  PLISSIT model, 57–85, 123, 177, 185
  and sexual rehabilitation, 123
bibliotherapy, 72
bisexuality, 33, 44, 133, 161, 163, 167, 178
  and AIDS, 103–4
  in children and adolescents, 199, 201
  married men, 94
  in women, 27–8, 163
  see also homosexuality; lesbian relationships;
    sexual orientation concerns;
    transgenderism
body image, 122, 123, 124, 195–6, 202, 205
body language of practitioner, 14–15, 23, 25,
  26, 30, 54
brachioproctic sexual practices and STDs, 46
breast cancer, 3, 113, 116–17, 211, 212

Cass's stages of homosexual adjustment, 90–111,
  167–8
cervical cancer, 3, 115
children
  behavioral problems, 185–8, 194–5, 196–9
  body image, 195–6, 202
  homosexuality, 199–203
  legal considerations in treating, 158, 190,
    191, 192
  parent–child counselling, 186–8
  parental concerns, 185–6
  paraphilias, 196–9
  practitioner–patient language, 15, 23, 182,
    187
  sexual abuse, 190–4
  sexual counselling, 182–203
  and sexual history taking, 8, 182–4, 186–8,
    197
  and sexual learning, 185–6
chlamydia, 1, 116, 139, 157
chronic illness and sexuality, 120–5, 206–8
Coleman's stages of homosexual identity
  development, 95, 167, 168
compulsive sexual behavior, 63, 64–5
  and HIV/AIDS, 99, 108, 141
  impact on daily life, 64–5
  object insertion, 118
  treatment, 65
condoms
  contraception, 46–7, 190
  effect on ejaculation and erection, 98, 114
  female condom, 98, 114–15
  prophylactic history, 12
  STD prevention, 3, 46–7, 98, 114–15, 134,
    136, 137–8, 189
  to treat premature ejaculation, 73
  use by homosexual men, 91
confidentiality, 14, 41–2, 52, 139, 151–2,
  157–8, 193, 202
contact tracing for STDs see partner
  notification
context in sexual history taking, 8–9
contraception, 3, 12, 47, 113–14, 127, 189–90
  see also condoms
couples therapy, 52–3, 63, 70–3, 74–5, 77–80
  and chronic illness, 122, 123–4
  and confidentiality, 151–2
  see also behavioral counselling; sensate focus
    exercises

cross-dressing *see* transgenderism
cultural factors, 8, 89

depression
  and HIV/AIDS, 98, 104, 135, 136, 144, 147
  loss of libido, 122
  and relationship problems, 13
  resulting from STDs, 87, 88, 90, 102, 135
  and sexual identity, 168
  and unprotected sex, 98
diabetic neuropathy, 35, 38
drugs
  and HIV/AIDS risk, 98, 128, 136, 138, 140
  safe needle use, 136, 138, 140
  sexual function and drug abuse, 13, 118, 122, 128
  and unsafe sex, 118–19, 128
  see also individual drug names; medication
dry ejaculation, 74, 214–15
dyspareunia, 39
dysphoria
  gender, 178–9
  and STDs, 93–4
  see also sexual orientation concerns

ejaculation *see* dry ejaculation; premature
    ejaculation; retarded ejaculation
elderly *see* older patient
empathy in practitioner–patient
    communication, 16–17, 51, 54, 55
erectile dysfunction, 3, 4, 30, 35, 66–8
  aging and, 205, 212–13
  alcohol and, 126–7
  cannabis and, 128
  caused by medication, 58, 74, 75, 127–8, 213
  chemical interventions, 66–8
  and condom use, 98
  primary, 35
  and retarded ejaculation, 74, 75
  secondary, 35
  sensate focus exercises, 66
  Viagra, 1, 3, 66–8, 73
ethical considerations, 151–60
  see also legal considerations; value judgments
    by practitioner

gay bowel syndrome, 174
gender identity, 60, 162, 178–9, 186, 188
  see also transgenderism
genital herpes *see* herpes
genital warts *see* human papilloma virus
Goldman's Rule, 15–16, 23
gonorrhea, 1, 39, 116, 139, 157, 174

heart attack and sexual activity, 122, 207–8
hepatitis (A, B, C), 1, 96, 139, 174
herpes, 1, 40, 96, 101–2
  and cancer, 115
  counselling for, 97, 101–2, 130–49
  diagnostic testing for, 130–3
  effects on lifestyle, 101–2

and homosexual men, 174
preventive education, 136–7, 147–8
problems with history taking, 43
reactions to diagnosis, 103–7, 134–5, 143, 147, 148
recurrence, 101
risk behaviors, 133–4, 136, 140–1
seen as 'punishment', 91
and sexual dysfunction, 102–3
stigmatization, 135, 136–7, 144
treatment, 146–8
see also sexually transmissible diseases (STDs)
herpes simplex infection *see* herpes
HIV/AIDS, 1, 40
  AIDS phobias, 91–3, 94, 133, 141
  counselling for, 87, 91–3, 94, 96, 97, 98, 103–9, 111, 130–49
  and genital warts, 115–16
  giving patient negative/positive results, 140–5
  and homosexual men, 174
  legal considerations in treating, 1, 157–8, 159
  negative consequences, discussion of, 136–7
  patient education, 136–7, 147–8, 188
  patient empowerment, 107
  primary prevention, 137–8, 140–1, 147–8
  problems with history taking, 43
  reaction to diagnosis, 103–9, 134–5, 143, 147, 148
  risk factors, 41, 98–9, 128, 133–4, 140–1, 155, 188
  seen as 'punishment', 91
  stigmatization, 103–4, 110, 111, 135, 136–7, 144, 154, 162
  testing, 93, 130–49, 159
  treatment, 145, 146–8
  see also sexually transmissible diseases (STDs)
homophobia, internalized *see* homosexuality—
    denial of
homosexuality, 161–79
  Cass's stages of homosexual adjustment, 90–111, 167–8
  in children and adolescents, 188, 199–203
  Coleman's stages of homosexual identity
    development, 95, 167, 168
  coming out, 105, 167, 168, 170–1, 176–8, 200, 201
  denial of, 90–1, 94, 110, 164, 168–9, 170–1, 175–6, 201
  homosexual males and STDs, 90–111, 137, 138, 161, 170, 174
  lesbian relationships, 27–8, 79–80, 161–79
  in married men, 93–4, 177
  and psychosomatic illness, 170–1
  relationship profiles, 171–3
  and sexual history taking, 24, 26, 27, 33, 44
  statistics, 133, 161, 162, 163, 199, 200
  and STDs, 87–111, 161, 170–1, 173–5
  stigmatization of, 90, 94–5, 104, 161–2, 164
  see also bisexuality; transgenderism
hormone replacement therapy, 210
hormones and sexual function 126–8, 205, 209–11, 212

human immunodeficiency virus (HIV) see
    HIV/AIDS
human papilloma virus, 1, 115–16
hypoactive sexual desire, 35, 63–4
hypothyroidism, 64

iatrogenic factors in sexual dysfunction see
    medication
impotence, 74
incest, 192, 193
infertility, 27, 39, 81–5
insomnia, 13
intensive therapy in sexual counselling, 59

Kegel exercises, 59, 70
Kinsey's Rule, 15, 24

language in practitioner–patient
    communication, 15–16, 23–4, 33, 144,
    170, 182, 187, 203
legal considerations, 151–60
    children and adolescents, 8, 158, 190, 191,
        192
    criminal law, 158
    and HIV/AIDS counselling, 1, 130, 136,
        157–8
    and partner notification of STDs, 48–9
    and patient confidentiality, 41, 151, 157–8,
        193, 202
    and practitioner–patient relationship, 152,
        159
lesbian relationships, 27–8, 79–80, 161–79
    lesbian children and adolescents, 188,
        199–203
    sexual health care, 174–5
    see also bisexuality; homosexuality;
        transgenderism
limited information in sexual counselling, 58

manual sex and STDs, 45–6
masturbation
    and anorgasmia, 75–7
    and bereavement and separation, 208–9
    children and, 185, 186
    and compulsive sexual behavior, 65
    and HIV/AIDS, 108
    normalizing approach, 33
    and premature ejaculation, 70
    and retarded ejaculation, 74, 75
    after sensate focus exercises, 70
    and STDs, 4–5
medication, 126–9
    chemotherapy, 123
    and dry ejaculation, 74
    and erectile problems, 58, 213
    patient education for use of, 97
    and prescription of Viagra, 67–8, 73
    and retarded ejaculation, 73–4, 127
    and sexual problems, 38, 58–9, 64, 73, 120,
        122, 123
    and STDs, 40–1, 128
    taking a history of, 40

    to treat HIV/AIDS, 146, 147
    to treat paraphilias, 197
    to treat premature ejaculation, 73
menopause/post-menopause, 128, 205, 209–11
minors see adolescents; children; legal
    considerations
Mitford's Rule, 16
multiple sclerosis, 38
'My week, your week' exercise, 63

neurological damage, 35, 38
nitrites, volatile, 67, 68, 118, 128
non-gonococcal urethritis, 174
non-penetrative sexual practices and STDS,
    46–7

obstetric history, 25–6
older patient, 205–15
    bereavement and separation, 208–9
    chronic illness or injury, 206–8
    menopause/post-menopause, 128, 205,
        209–11
    prostate problems, 38, 113, 117, 124,
        213–15
    and retarded ejaculation, 74, 212
    retirement, 205–6
    and sexual history taking, 8
oral sex and STDs, 45
orgasmic dysfunction, 35, 60, 74, 75–80,
    214–15
    see also anorgasmia
Orwell's Rule, 16, 23

Pap smear, 3, 10, 113, 114, 212
paraphilias, 60, 65, 186, 196–9
partner notification of STDs, 41, 48–9, 88, 94,
    100
patient education
    and adolescents, 188–9
    and children, 185–6
    and HIV/AIDS, 136–7, 148
    and homosexuality, 176
    and premature ejaculation, 72
    preventive health care, 3, 12, 40, 41, 50,
        97–100, 113–19, 132, 133, 136, 137–8,
        140–1, 147–8, 154, 157, 188–9
pelvic inflammatory disease, 3, 116
permission in sexual counselling, 57
Peyronie's disease, 39, 213
pharmacotherapy see medication
phobias see HIV/AIDS—AIDS phobias;
    venerophobias
PLISSIT model of sexual counselling, 57–85,
    123, 177, 184, 185 poppers see nitrites,
    volatile
practitioner–patient relationship, improper, 152,
    159
pregnancy, 10, 26
    see also contraception; infertility; obstetric
        history
premature ejaculation, 4, 33, 35, 36–7, 68–73
    behavioral treatment, 69–73

sensate focus exercises, 60–2, 73
squeeze technique, 59
preventive health care, 3, 12, 40, 41, 50,
    97–100, 108–9, 113–19, 132, 133, 136,
    137–8, 140–1, 147–8, 154, 157, 188–9
    see also individual diseases; condoms; drugs;
    patient education; safe/safer sex
primary prevention *see* individual diseases;
    patient education; preventive health care
priapism *see* prolonged penile erection
prolactin secretion, increased, 127
prolonged penile erection, 68
prophylactic practice *see* condoms; preventive
    health care
prostate problems
    cancer, 117, 213–5
    conducting examinations for, 113, 214
    surgery, 38, 214–15
psychiatric disorders and sexuality, 120–2
public health considerations, 154–6, 157–8

rehabilitation, sexual, 123–4
relationships
    bereavement and separation, 208–9
    and chronic illness, 122–4, 206–8
    and disclosure of patient information, 157
    effects of retirement, 205–6
    history taking, 31, 33–4
    homosexual, 171–3
    infertility and, 81–5
    married men and homosexuality, 93–4, 177
    masturbation with partner 75, 77–8
    older patient, 205–9
    partner focus, 72
    practitioner–patient, improper, 152, 159
    problems caused by STDs, 88, 93, 104
    and sexual problems, 13, 14, 26–7, 28–31,
        33–4, 52–3, 68, 74
    structure, 26–7
    Viagra's effects on, 68
    see also couples therapy; sexual desire
        discrepancy
retarded ejaculation, 35, 37–9, 60, 73–5, 81,
    127
retrograde ejaculation, 74, 214–15
role play for practitioner
    for sexual history taking, 17, 20
    for giving HIV/AIDS test results, 142

safe/safer-sex practices *see* condoms; drugs;
    patient education; preventive health care
schizophrenia and sexuality, 122
screening history, 10–12, 13
self-actualization, 51
Semans' technique, 70–2
sensate focus exercises, 59, 60–2, 66, 70–2, 73,
    77–9
setting of interview/counselling, 14–15, 23,
    54
sex therapist, referral to, 59, 74, 80, 138
sex toys, 46, 113, 117–18
sexual abuse, 9, 24, 98

of children and adolescents, 190–4, 201
law regarding, 158, 190, 191, 192
sexual aversion disorder, 63–4
sexual counselling
    general theory and practice, 51–4
    PLISSIT model, 57–85, 123, 177, 184, 185
sexual desire discrepancy, 63
sexual disorders, categories of, 60
sexual dysfunction, 2, 28–31, 35–9
    and herpes, 102–3
    medication and, 126–9
    PLISSIT model of sexual counselling for,
        57–85
    prevalence of, 3–4
    screening history for, 10–11
    specific to men, 35–9
    specific to women, 28–31
    treatment, 60–80
    see also individual dysfunctions
sexual history taking, 1–50
    from children and adolescents, 7–8, 15, 23,
        24, 182–4, 186–8, 197
    confidentiality, 158
    context, 8–9
    and couples therapy, 53
    cultural differences, 8
    difficulties in, 5–6
    drug-use history, 129
    empathy in, 16–17
    explaining rationale to patient, 17
    full medical history, 7, 12, 13
    gender differences, 8, 24–39
    homosexuality and, 24, 26, 27, 33, 44
    identifying the need for, 7–10
    and infertility, 82–3
    and intellectual handicap, 10
    language in, 15, 23–4, 187
    legal considerations, 8, 41, 48–9, 152, 158,
        159
    location of, 14–15, 23, 54
    male-specific, 32–9
    patient consent, 153
    practice in, 17, 21
    reasons for, 10–12
    for relationship difficulties, 13
    for screening, 10
    for sexual dysfunction, 10–11, 28–31, 35–9,
        64, 70
    for sexual practices, 44–6
    skill in, 2–4
    for STDs, 6, 40–50
    timing of, 10–12
    value judgments and, 9, 10, 15, 20, 21
    woman-specific, 3, 10–11, 24–32
sexual identity, 162–3, 166–8
sexual orientation concerns, 161–79, 188, 199,
    200–3
    see also bisexuality; homosexuality; sexual
        identity; transgenderism
sexual practices
    STDs and, 173
    taking a history of, 44–6

sexual reorientation, 168–9
sexually transmissible diseases (STDs), 1,
   87–111
   abnormal illness behaviors, 109–10
   acceptance of, 95–6
   adolescents, 188–9
   attributions of, 89
   and cancer of lower genital tract, 115
   compliance with treatment, 89, 97, 109
   confidentiality, 41–2, 139, 157–8
   counselling for, 87–111, 130–49
   definition, 40
   diagnostic testing, 130–3
   ethical considerations, 154–6
   as evidence of maladjustment, 93–4
   as fault of sick society, 94–5, 96
   government notification, 41, 156–7
   homosexuality and, 87–111, 161, 170–1,
      173–5
   legal considerations in treating, 130, 136
   and medication, 40–1, 128
   partner notification, 41, 48–9, 88, 94, 100
   and patient education, 40, 50, 88, 97–100,
      136–7, 188–9
   preventing disease transmission, 46–7,
      97–100, 114–15, 132, 133, 136–8, 147–8,
      154, 157, 189
   psychological effects, 88–111, 132, 134–5
   risk factors, 44–6, 98–9, 132, 140–1, 155,
      173, 174, 189
   screening, 130–3
   seen as 'punishment', 88, 90–2
   sexual history taking for, 6, 40–50
   as source of pride, 96
   stigmatization, 41, 87, 88, 90, 94–5, 109,
      136–7, 154
   testing for, 130–9
   see also hepatitis (A, B, C); herpes;
      HIV/AIDS; syphilis
sexually transmitted diseases
   definition, 40
   see also gonorrhea; human papilloma virus
specific suggestions in sexual counselling, 59
spectatoring, 62, 66, 77
spinal cord injury, 123–4
squeeze technique, 59, 70
stress, sex used to cope with, 108
stroke and sexual activity, 122, 207–8
suicide risk, 144, 147, 168, 192
   as a response to herpes or HIV diagnosis,
      105, 135
   and homosexuality, 91
   adolescent, 200–2, 203
syphilis, 1, 89, 139, 157

testicular cancer, 3, 113, 117
testosterone levels and aging, 212–13

therapist skills, 53–5
transgenderism, 178–9, 188, 199
   see also gender identity

unsafe sex, 108–9, 133–4, 136
   see also alcohol; depression; drugs; herpes;
      HIV/AIDS; patient education; preventive
      health care; safe/safer sex; sexually
      transmissible diseases (STDs)
urethra, problems of the, 39, 45
uterine cancer, 212

vaginal atrophy, 210
vaginal intercourse and STDs, 45
vaginal lubrication, oestrogens and, 128
vaginismus, 30–1, 80–1
value judgments by practitioner
   in assisting with sexual orientation concerns,
      176–7
   in sexual history taking, 9, 10, 15, 20, 21
   in treating STDs, 100–1, 161–2
venerophobias, 91–3, 109, 133, 141
Viagra, 1, 3, 66–8, 73

women, specific considerations
   anorgasmia, 27, 28–9, 35, 36, 75–80
   bisexuality, 27–8, 163
   breast cancer, 3, 113, 116–17, 211, 212
   cervical cancer, 3, 115
   contraception, 3, 12, 47, 113–14, 127,
      189–90
   female condom, 98, 114–15
   gynaecological problems, 10
   hormone replacement therapy, 210
   infertility, 27, 39, 81–5
   intercourse history, 26
   lesbian relationships, 27–8, 79–80, 161–79,
      188, 199–203
   menopause/post-menopause, 128, 205,
      209–11
   menstrual history, 24
   obstetric history, 25
   oestrogens, 128, 210
   older women, 205–12
   orgasmic dysfunction, 35, 60, 74, 75–80,
      214–15
   Pap smear, 3, 10, 113, 114, 212
   pelvic inflammatory disease, 3, 116
   pregnancy, 10, 26
   screening history, 10–11
   sexual dysfunction, 4, 27, 28–31, 75–85
   sexual history taking, 3, 10–11, 24–32
   sexual self-image and chronic illness, 123,
      124
   STDs, 10, 174–5
   uterine cancer, 212

SETON HALL UNIVERSITY
UNIVERSITY LIBRARIES
SO. ORANGE, NJ 07079-2671